D0391312

Praise for *Diabetes Do's & How-To's*

"*Diabetes Do's & How-To's* is such a fun, informative, and unique way to help you take control of your diabetes."
— Steven Edelman, MD, Founder and Director of Taking Control of Your Diabetes

"As a PWD and a CDE, we **need** more books like *Diabetes Do's & How-To's*. It gets right to the point of solving problems that we deal with day in and day out…who could (or should) ask for more?"
— Gary Scheiner, MS, CDE, Integrated Diabetes Services, and author of *Think Like A Pancreas*

"*Diabetes Do's & How-To's* provides goals with guts—which sets this book apart from, and above, the many other resources for persons with diabetes. It's a road map for persons and families living with diabetes…it gives you short cuts, and helps you find your way around mountains. Riva Greenberg takes the "Do's"—the goals frequently given to persons with diabetes—and translates them into practical steps for implementing in real life. Realistic and simple, without ever being simplistic…the author's compassionate, humorous and championing voice is complemented by the wickedly insightful drawings of Haidee Merritt."
— Barbara J. Anderson, PhD, Professor of Pediatrics, Associate Head of Psychology, Baylor College of Medicine

"This latest book by Riva Greenberg is brimming with practical and useful advice for the person with any type of diabetes or anyone who wants to avoid type 2. It makes effective diabetes management simple and attainable."
— Sheri Colberg, PhD, expert on diabetes and exercise, and author of eight books

DISCARD

"Riva Greenberg has written a terrific book, filled with practical and clinically sound wisdom that's been turned into clear and vital action steps. Riva conveys optimism and inspires motivation through her lighthearted voice and anecdotes about her personal trials enacting her own advice. *Diabetes Do's & How-To's* deserves to be a key resource for anyone who has, or wishes to prevent, diabetes, and for physicians and dietitians to distribute widely."
— Terry Stein, MD, Internal Medicine

"Although I am a physician, I wish that I had a book like this when I started my journey with diabetes over forty years ago."
— Lawrence Gottlieb, MD

"*Diabetes Do's & How-To's* is packed with something missing from most diabetes books: advice that you can actually use to improve your life. Greenberg paints a path toward a fulfilling, energizing life with diabetes."
— David Edelman, President and Co-Founder of DiabetesDaily.com

"WOW!!! Having lived with diabetes for thirty years...this book breaks it down, step by step, and helps you get on top. Riva is a magician, and her words will help you and your family fulfill all your dreams with diabetes!"
— Phil Southerland, Founder/CEO Team Type 1, and author of *Not Dead Yet*

"A delightful spin on diabetes self-care by focusing on things that you CAN do...here is a refreshing perspective on diabetes, which is all too often seen as a disease of don'ts."
— Claire Blum, MS Ed, RN, CDE, living with diabetes for thirty-four-plus years

"Riva Greenberg's third book fills a huge void for us—the "how-to's" most books leave us longing for, and inspiration that is genuine, humorous, heart-felt, and much-needed. As someone with diabetes, and a wellness coach working with clients who have diabetes, this is *the* diabetes primer—both for patients and busy health care providers."
— Heather Nielsen, MA, counselor and wellness coach

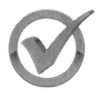

Diabetes Do's
& How-To's

SMALL YET POWERFUL STEPS TO TAKE CHARGE,
EAT RIGHT, GET FIT, AND STAY POSITIVE

Riva Greenberg

SPI Management LLC
Brooklyn, New York

Riva Greenberg is the author of *50 Diabetes Myths That Can Ruin Your Life and the 50 Diabetes Truths That Can Save It* and *The ABC's Of Loving Yourself With Diabetes*.

SPI Management, L.L.C.
Brooklyn, New York 11215

Copyright ©2013 by Riva Greenberg
Illustrations ©2013 Haidee Merritt

All rights reserved. No part of this book may be reproduced in whole or in part without written permission by the author, except by reviewers, who may quote brief excerpts in connection with a review in a newspaper, magazine, or electronic publication; nor may any part of this book be reproduced, stored in a retrieval system or transmitted in any form or by any means, electronic or mechanical, including duplication, recording, or other, without the prior written permission of the author.

The information in this book is true and complete to the best of our knowledge. This book is intended only as an informative guide for those wishing to know more about health issues. In no way is this book intended to replace, countermand, or conflict with the advice given to you by your own physician. The ultimate decision concerning care should be made between you and your doctor. We strongly recommend you follow his or her advice. Information in this book is general and is offered with no guarantees on the part of the author and contributors. The author and publisher disclaim all liability in connection with the use of this book. Also, while I recommend various products in the book, I have neither been asked to, nor compensated for, doing so.

ISBN: 978-0-9822906-1-3

Library of Congress Control Number: 2012914925

First edition 2013
Printed in the United States of America

Text by Riva Greenberg
Cartoons by Haidee S. Merritt
Editing by Gary Feit
Cover and interior design by Bill Greaves

This book is available at special quantity discounts, and to use as premiums and sales promotions. For more information, please go to: diabetesbydesign.com/publications.

Come to the edge
No, I can't, I might fall!
Come to the edge
No, I can't, it's too far!
Come to the edge
No, I can't, it's too high!
COME TO THE EDGE!
And so, I came,
He pushed me,
and I flew!

When we are about to make a change in our lives, we often feel afraid. Yet I know that with hope, and the desire to live your best life, you can. I also know you have the power within you, and around you, to help you fly.

This poem is an adaptation, made by my friend Jill Hughes, of Christopher Logue's poem, "Come to the Edge."

Table of Contents

Bonus Do's 217

As you begin working with a "Do,"
put a mark in the box next to it.
When you feel you've made significant progress,
you can check that "Do" off the list.

Major Contributing Experts

Sandy Merrill, MPH, CHHC. Nutrition & Wellness Coach in private practice in Manhattan helping people with diabetes and pre-diabetes recover their health through healthy eating and lifestyle changes. Website: www.sandymerrill.com.

Lynda Schultz Sardeson, MSA, RN, CDE, PWD. Past President of the Northern Indiana Association of Diabetes Educators, National and International Certified Diabetes Educator.

Kathy Spain, RN, BSN, CDE, CPT. Founder of Diabetes Consulting Network, Certified Diabetes Educator, and past member of JDRF's Research Lay Review Committee.

Susan Weiner, RD, MS, CDE, CDN. Registered Dietitian and Certified Diabetes Educator in private practice in New York. Contributing Medical Producer for dLife TV and a member of dLife's medical advisory board. Top 10 Nutrition Educator blogger. Website: www.susanweiner nutrition.com.

Delaine M. Wright, MS, CEP, CDE. Masters level Clinical Exercise Physiologist, Certified Diabetes Educator and Pump/CGM Trainer. Team Leader/Program Coordinator, Cardiac Rehab and Wellness at South County Hospital in Wakefield, RI.

Message from Dr. Michael Dansinger

Weight Loss and Nutrition Adviser for TV's *The Biggest Loser*
and Director of the Diabetes Reversal Program, Tufts University School of Medicine

Congratulations! The fact that you are reading the words on this page means that you are seriously interested in creating your best possible life—yes, even with diabetes. And even if you have pre-diabetes or your doctor has told you that your blood sugar is borderline.

Can diabetes be a blessing rather than a curse? Yes, it can. Not only can you thrive in spite of your diabetes, but you can enjoy a richer, more fulfilling life because of it. With Riva Greenberg's expert guidance, you can dramatically speed up the process of transforming both your diabetes and your life for the better. Millions have and you can too.

To do so, you'll need to learn *how* to manage your diabetes, and that's what this book is all about. It gives you the essential steps you need to take to help you optimize your diabetes health. Knowing what to do, and how to do it, may be just what you've been missing in your attempt to manage your diabetes.

The same is true for pre-diabetes. Most of these steps will help you turn around your health so you may never get diabetes. Pre-diabetes means you're headed in the direction of type 2 diabetes, but we know that by eating healthier, losing a little weight, and getting a little more active, you can prevent type 2 diabetes or delay its onset.

The truth is, people with diabetes and pre-diabetes don't get into trouble because they don't try. The problem is that so much information is out there, and it's very confusing to know what to do. Chances are no one has spent enough time helping you understand just what to do and how to do it.

To maximize your diabetes health, you need good information and you need it to be easy to understand and follow so you can use it right now. That's what you now have. Bite-sized action steps for healthy eating, getting more activity into your day, monitoring your blood sugar (and what to do with the numbers), preventing diabetes complications, working with your medical team, and dealing with the many other aspects of diabetes. If you have pre-diabetes, you need to do many of the things in this book, too, and keep a watch on your blood sugar and discuss with your doctor if you should be on a medication now that can keep your blood sugar from rising.

But Riva has put together not just *what* you need to do, but also suggestions on *how* to do it. Riva, who has had diabetes for four decades, knows that it takes more than knowledge to live successfully with diabetes. It takes a *success system* that guarantees you make good decisions and can follow through with appropriate actions. The information and concepts presented here, Riva and I both know, create that success system that you need for managing your diabetes and transforming your life.

I also know that when you begin to consistently nourish your body with the right nutrients, challenge your muscles with the right amount of exercise, and feel a fire in your belly to do whatever it takes to be healthy and well, you strengthen your body, mind, spirit, and self-control. You charge and ready yourself for success, in your diabetes health and in every aspect of your life.

Now I ask you to bring your emotional commitment and personal passion to taking action, and know with every fiber of your being that you deserve to live a full, productive, and joyful life with diabetes.

I couldn't be happier that you have found this book. Taking back your power by following the steps in this book is the key to truly having the best control of your diabetes and starting to live life to the fullest.

I wish you great success and excellent health for years to come!

Sincerely,

Michael Dansinger, MD

Note to My Readers

Welcome. I'm so happy you've found this book. Whether you or a family member has diabetes, I am excited that you now have a tool that provides the specific actions to take to help you or a loved one start living a healthier, happier life.

While the "Do's" and "How-To's" in this book lean a bit more toward type 2 diabetes, no matter what type of diabetes you have (including type 1, LADA, and gestational diabetes), you'll find information here to benefit you. If you have pre-diabetes (blood sugar levels that are higher than normal but not yet high enough to be diagnosed as type 2 diabetes), as nearly 80 million Americans do, pay particular attention to the "Do's" about eating healthy foods, maintaining a healthy weight, getting physically active now, working with your doctor, and understanding your lab tests. These and many of the other "Do's" in this book may help you prevent ever getting diabetes or delay its onset. (If you don't know what type of diabetes you have, see "What Diabetes Is—and Why it's Confusing" on page 236.)

If you are a health care professional and work with people who have diabetes, this book can help you guide your patients to take small powerful steps to better manage their diabetes. You'll find a tool to use with your patients on the page "For Health Care Professionals: How to Work More Effectively with Patients."

Why I Wrote This Book

So often when I travel across the US and to other countries to speak to people with diabetes, this is what I hear: "Can I eat fried chicken?" "What's the best thing to have for breakfast?" "My blood sugar's fine in the morning, why is my doctor telling me to take another pill?" I hear confusion, which is understandable because diabetes is a complex, chronic condition that we patients, not our doctors, have to manage. I also see that the vast majority of people—people everywhere and from all walks of life—who have trouble managing their diabetes aren't lazy or unmotivated; rather, they simply don't know what to do—and how to do it.

I wrote this book to answer the urgent need all of us who live with diabetes have for simple, clear information about what to do to take care of our diabetes and how to do it. While you may spend up to a dozen hours with your health care providers each year, you spend more than 8,700 hours on your own, making daily decisions that affect your diabetes.

The information and steps here provide you with the ability to make smart and healthful decisions. You will know now what nourishing foods to eat and how much, how to bring your weight within a normal range if necessary, how to get more physical activity, how to take your medicines on time and as prescribed, how to de-stress, and how to shift your mindset from "overwhelmed" to "unshakable confidence." Now you can begin to live a life of greater health, with more energy, enjoyment, calm, capability, and happiness.

About This Book

These "Do's" and "How-To's" are collected from leading health professionals in diabetes and my own forty years of experience living with diabetes. While my journey with diabetes had a rocky start, by doing much of what I suggest in this book, I am now in the best health I can imagine for myself. I have reduced my weight from my high of 165 pounds to the weight I maintain today, 127 pounds. Each time I go for my lab tests, my results are remarkably good. I walk an hour a day, gladly, because it keeps me strong and increases my insulin sensitivity. And, following the action steps I share with you in this book, I am committed and able to keep myself well.

I learned some new things writing this book, so even though I've had diabetes for forty years and manage it extremely well, there is always something new and useful to learn. For instance, I learned more about what makes us fat and how to create a meal plan to keep from gaining weight. I learned why it's important to remove your insulin pen needle after each injection, and if you have retinopathy (diabetic eye disease), why you should check with your doctor before starting any anaerobic (intense, strength-based, gasping-for-air) exercise.

How to Approach Taking a New Action

You should know that not all the explanations of the "Do's" are academically or scientifically complete. Making them so would have made the text so complicated at times that it may have further confused or discouraged you from taking action. So for our purposes in this book, the explanations are complete enough to understand why the "Do" is important and to easily take an action. To put it another way, we don't have to know how an engine works to drive a car. If we did, most of us would be sitting at home—at least I know I would.

Here's the best way to look at taking a new action: if you apply a "How-To" from this book today, then you have made today a little bit better than yesterday. Give yourself a pat on the back. As you're ready, take another small step forward so that tomorrow will be a little bit better than today. With each step forward, congratulate yourself for your effort. When I was finishing this book, I was on a flight to Indianapolis where I sat next to a young man whose T-shirt captivated me. On the back it said, "Tomorrow's battle is won during today's practice." I can't think of a better way to say that every step we take now benefits us for the years to come.

You should also know the actions I suggest here are not merely good advice; rather, they are what works in real life, and they will change your life. In the end, if you have diabetes or pre-diabetes, it doesn't have to determine how healthy you can be. We know today that our actions, not our genetics, are as responsible for determining our health, if not more so.

How to Use This Book

Before you dive in, reading the following will help you get the most out of this book. Also know that much of what you read here may hold true

xvi | DIABETES DO'S & HOW-TO'S

for the majority of people with diabetes, but it may be somewhat different for you. We are all different and our bodies work differently. Always talk to your doctor before you make any changes to your treatment plan. Also, by working hand-in-hand with your health care providers, you'll be able to use these steps to your best personal advantage.

This book is, as Dr. Dansinger says, a *"success system."* It is a guide to make smart and wise decisions, to follow through with the actions that support those decisions, to take the best care of yourself, and to live your best life with diabetes.

The "Do's" in this book cover four categories: food, medicine, exercise, and attitude. At the end of each "Do" are suggestions called "How-To's" that explain how to put these "Do's" into action. You may want to skim through the whole book to get familiar with what's here, or go directly to a "Do" you're curious about or want to start working on. Or you may want to read the section "What Diabetes Is—and Why it's Confusing" first for an overview of diabetes. There is no order to go in and there is no pace to go at. Starting anywhere, and taking one small step, will improve your diabetes and your health.

Quick-Starts

There are two Quick-Starts at the end of each "Do." These are relatively fast and easy steps you can take to do a "Do." Starting with a Quick-Start is a way to jump start your success and build your confidence.

How-To's

Following each Quick-Start is a list of "How-To's." I don't by any means intend for you to do all these things. These "How-To's" provide you suggestions to choose from. See what appeals to you, what you think you can do, and what you are willing to do. The most important thing is to pick something you feel you can do and make a small start. You can accomplish great things with small steps.

Be aware, however, that doing too much at once is the fastest way to fail. You will feel overwhelmed, frustrated, defeated, or burned out.

Most of us are better able to make and sustain changes when we take small steps and experience success. My suggestion is to start with just one or two "How-To's" for one or two "Do's." When you've mastered them, or if you find you're not ready to take on what you chose, make a new or different choice.

Worksheets and Other Thoughts

Worksheets are provided at the end of each category, and there is one in the back of the book that you can make copies of. These worksheets are simple tools for you to make a simple start on taking action. They are based on some of the latest insights about how people make lasting changes in their lives. Use them to write down what you are going to work on, and think through the specifics of how you will do it. Also, feel free to come up with your own "How-To's." These can be just as powerful as what's offered here.

I encourage you to see the actions you will take as "experiments." Meaning, try something, have an open and curious mind about it, and see what happens. When you "experiment" you can't fail, you can only learn from the results of your experiment.

The end of each category also includes tips from fellow patients. In addition to learning from our doctors, we also learn from each other. I hope their tips and stories will help you feel less alone, and inspire you to take action. Then with all you learn here, you will inspire others.

I refer to our medical professionals by different names—doctor, health care provider, physician, general practitioner—only to keep from repeating myself. That said, a diabetes educator is different. That is someone specifically trained in diabetes and the care of people with diabetes.

Lastly, as you read through and work with this book, use Haidee Merritt's cartoons as a rest stop. Pause and have a laugh when you get to them. I included Haidee's cartoons not because diabetes is a joke, but because her keen wit tells a bit of our universal story of living with diabetes, and she makes me laugh. And laughter, along with being forgiving and kind with ourselves, is essential to keep going when we tire of the work of diabetes.

For Health Care Professionals

Working with your patients on the worksheets can help you, together, discover their strengths, and turn on their thinking and desire to make healthy behavior changes. On page 233 are strategies you can use, and targeted questions you can ask your patients, based on the latest insights in neuroscience and positive psychology. They will make both of you more successful.

Final Thoughts For Your Success

Share this book with family and friends, particularly when you are working on a "Do." Think how they might support you. Also, bring this book to your health care professionals and let them know what you'd like to work on. They can help guide and support you by personalizing what's here for your particular needs. Individualized treatment plans and goals are so important that the American Diabetes Association made them an official recommendation for health care providers this year.

Lastly, I hope this book will get opened, put aside, opened, thrown on the coffee table, lost under the couch, found again, get coffee spilled on it, get closed, and opened again. I hope it will serve you as a trusted friend and resource—an owner's manual of sorts—that you will return to again and again. And, as you work with it, you will find your diabetes is easier to manage, your health improves, and you begin to live the life you deserve—one that is full, rich, productive, healthy, and happy. Living these "Do's" has changed my health and my life for the better. I wish the same for you.

YOU'RE STRONG (enough)

(Hold under chin while looking in mirror)

Food Note

It's not surprising if you're confused about how to eat healthy. Every day we hear new reports and new recommendations, many of which contradict each other. Even experts within the diabetes and dietitian communities have different points of view about how we should eat. For instance: low-carb or high-carb? Low-fat or full-fat? Should we avoid saturated fat completely?

The "Food Do's" in this book reflect current conventional wisdom and health guidelines. They mirror the recommendations of most health care providers and dietitians. Where I felt it important, they also give experts' thinking who differ in opinion, as well as my own.

It's also important to remember that how food works in our body varies from person to person—something that raises my blood sugar a lot may not do that to yours. Other factors are also at play when it comes to foods' impact on our blood sugar, like what combination of foods we eat, how active we are, and the medicine we take.

In the end, you have to see how food works in *your* body. The best way is by checking your blood sugar before you eat something and two hours after your first bite, and seeing whether your blood sugar rose or fell, and how much. If you're not certain how to interpret the number you get on your meter, discuss it with your health care provider.

I want to also tell you about an eating plan that I became aware of in my research for this book called the paleo diet. The paleo diet, based on eating like our earliest ancestors in paleolithic times, contains higher amounts of protein and fat and fewer carbohydrates than the current recommended American diet. Richard Bernstein, a diabetologist who wrote the classic book, *Diabetes Solution,* and other paleo and low-carb eating advocates, say that eating high quality fats, including saturated fat found in animals, is healthy and not the cause of obesity and heart disease. This is significant since most people with type 2 diabetes are overweight, and have great difficulty losing weight. Plus, two-thirds of people with type 2 diabetes die of cardiovascular problems.

Paleo enthusiasts believe that when we eat more carbohydrates than we burn for energy, our body stores them as fat, and that this is the primary cause of weight gain and related ills. Advocates of the paleo diet also say it promotes better overall health, healthier digestion, and enhanced immunity. They also say it reduces fat storage, blood sugar spikes after a meal, and insulin-resistance. Certainly advantages for anyone with diabetes.

The paleo diet consists of lean meat, fish, fowl, vegetables, eggs, fruit, high quality fats, nuts, and seeds. The meats and poultry are preferably organic and free-range, the produce organic and locally grown. Grains are off limits and many paleo eaters also eliminate or limit dairy, soy, beans, and legumes. For most people eating a strict paleo diet is quite difficult, yet moving toward a diet of more protein, more healthy fat, and fewer carbohydrates may well be a move in the right direction.

Personally, my eating plan falls between paleo and a low-carb diet. It differs from a paleo diet by including complex carbohydrates like oatmeal, and in limited amounts, whole grains and beans. This diet is what works best for me.

I discovered two good paleo websites if you want further information: Mark Sisson's Mark's Daily Apple at marksdailyapple.com and Loren Cordain's The Paleo Diet at thepaleodiet.com. If you want to give it a try, talk with your health care provider and/or a dietitian or nutritionist, particularly if you have any other health conditions. And, as with all things, explore what works best for you.

Food Do's

By choosing healthier foods, you're choosing a longer life—
and you can stop sneaking those candy bars!

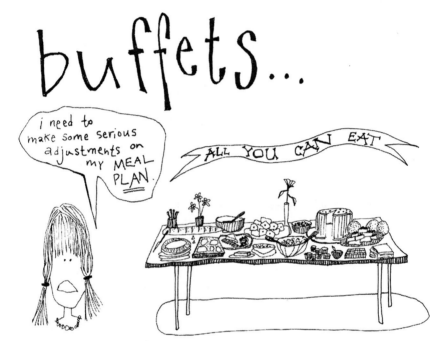

Do #1

Say "Bye-Bye" to Diets

If you've been on a diet, don't go on one again, ever. Really, I'm begging you! Diets are slippery slopes and usually only result in a temporary fix. As many as 83 percent of dieters gain back the weight they lose, and more. Plus, if you constantly try new diets, you actually end up tricking your metabolism and gaining weight, even when you eat fewer calories. Three decades ago I was thirty-five pounds heavier than I am today, and trust me, I dieted again and again, and it didn't work. Today I am about 127 pounds and I have maintained that weight for years. How did I get there and how do I maintain it? By eating mostly healthy foods, smaller portions, and walking an hour most days.

Carrying extra weight around your middle is particularly harmful because it can increase insulin-resistance—a condition people with type 2 diabetes have. It's when your body doesn't use the insulin it makes well enough for its needs. If your insulin resistance increases, you'll need more medicine to keep your blood sugar from rising too high. So losing some weight, if you need to, is a good thing. For many people, a small weight loss of 5–7 percent (typically ten to fifteen pounds) can help lower blood pressure, LDL (lousy) cholesterol, and triglycerides. And these are all risk factors for heart disease, which people with type 2 diabetes are three times more likely to suffer.

For some people with type 2 diabetes, losing some weight may reduce the amount of diabetes medicine you take, or eliminate it. The same is possible if you have pre-diabetes and you're taking medication. If you have type 1 diabetes and are overweight, losing some weight may reduce the amount of insulin you use and protect you from developing high blood pressure and high cholesterol. But diets aren't the answer. Even Weight Watchers says diets don't work. So stop dieting and start eating—healthy!

To lose weight *for good,* your eating habits must change *for life.* Like any member of a 12-step recovery program knows, lasting change is built on "one day at a time," each and every day.

Quick-Starts

☐ **Eat breakfast every morning.** Eating breakfast revs up your metabolism. If you skip breakfast you're likely to eat more calories by binging later in the day. In a study of people who lost weight and kept it off for more than five years, one major thing they all did was eat breakfast.

☐ **Familiarize yourself with proper portion sizes.** Read labels to see, and follow, single size portions for yourself and how much you need to make for your family. Use measuring cups or a food scale to see proper portion sizes. You won't need to do this forever, but doing it in the beginning helps you learn correct portion sizes.

Your Choice of More How-To's

☐ Don't get hung up on the numbers on the scale. A healthy lifestyle typically results in a healthy weight—so aim for health, make one healthier food choice each day. As you begin eating more nutritious foods and getting a little more physical activity (if you aren't physically active now), your body will come to its natural healthy weight.

☐ If you weigh yourself, I recommend doing it once a week, same day, same time, before breakfast, and know that your weight fluctuates a little. You might be retaining water or have just lost a pound from a bowel movement. I didn't own a scale for twenty-five years, I just went by how my clothes fit. Then three years ago my husband brought a scale into the house. After two years of just noticing it, now I weigh myself once a week. I use it as a guide to help me keep my weight where I want it to be, but I don't live or die with each weigh-in.

☐ Read through the healthy food choices in the "Food Do's" and look for foods to eat that are enjoyable and pleasing to you.

☐ Enlist family members and friends to eat healthier with you. It's easier when it's a team effort.

☐ Allow yourself to eat less healthy foods now and then, in small portions, unless there's a medical reason not to do so. Not letting yourself eat something you love may make you feel deprived and frustrated rather than excited about eating well.

☐ If you catch yourself gulping down cake or pie or a high calorie sweet without thinking, you have the opportunity to stop and think. Do you really need another bite or has your craving been satisfied? Don't throw away your good efforts just because you have a misstep. Eating half a piece of cake is better than eating the whole piece.

☐ Look for places in your day where you can cut down on, or cut out, one high calorie food you eat or drink. Replace a soda with a non-caloric drink, eat half a bagel or muffin, or skip your glazed jelly donut in the morning. Doing so adds up to weight lost each week, each month, each year. Slow but steady wins this race.

☐ Keep tempting foods out of the house and make them treats when you're out.

☐ Talk positively to yourself. Notice during the day what you're doing well to work toward your nutrition goals and compliment yourself. "Wow, you chose a healthy vegetable plate instead of a slice of pizza, great job!" The more you pat yourself on the back for what you're doing well, the more you'll inspire yourself to keep going. At the same time, quiet your inner critic. When you notice you're telling yourself you'll never succeed, or beating yourself up for having two bowls of ice cream, stop! A quick way to quiet your inner critic, and stop negative thoughts, is to move. Head out for a brief walk, turn on some music and sway, and above all, tell yourself tomorrow is a new day.

☐ When you notice you're thinking about food—which happens a lot when you're trying to lose, or watch your weight—shift your thoughts to something else. The less time you spend thinking about food, the less important you make it.

☐ If money motivates you, HealthyWage.com pays you to lose 10 percent of your weight and lets teams compete for up to $10,000. DietBet.com lets you bet against your friends. Those who reach their target weights by the last weigh-in win money.

Tips to create a healthy meal:

• Use the plate method, a simple formula for creating a healthy meal: Fill half your plate with low-carbohydrate vegetables like broccoli, green beans, zucchini, spinach, or cauliflower (you can also replace some vegetables with fruit). Fill one quarter of your plate with lean protein like grilled or baked fish, chicken, or pork. And fill one quarter of your plate with a whole grain or nutritious carbohydrate like brown rice, bulgur, barley, quinoa, or sweet potato.

• Learn, and eat in style, with these dishes that show you what foods to eat and how much: slimware.com and preciseportions.com.

• Fill up your plate in the kitchen and keep serving dishes off the table. It makes it easier not to take seconds. A Cornell University study showed that if you place a big bowl of pasta on the table, men eat 29 percent more and women eat 10 percent more than if you don't. I always fill my plate, once, in the kitchen. Of course I don't have a dining table, which helps!

• Serve dishes you love that are higher in fat and carbs, like macaroni and cheese, as side dishes instead of entrees.

• Replace sodas and fruit juices with water, or sparkling water with lemon or lime, or ice tea with low-calorie sweetener.

• Learn how to make smart food choices using this easy free app from EatSmart™. You'll get simple tips and tricks from noted dietitian and certified diabetes educator, Hope Warshaw, to achieve your diabetes "healthy meals" goals. Check it out at hopewarshaw.com/apps/eatsmart-hope-warshaw.

Tips to eat a healthy meal:

• Eat a salad before your meal (with lemon or vinegar and a little olive oil as dressing) or have a cup of broth and/or drink a glass of water. Not only is this healthy, it's also filling. You may eat a little less of your main meal.

• When you eat out, avoid buffets and all-you-can-eat deals at restaurants. It's too easy to overeat. Instead go to a restaurant where you can choose a healthy dish from the menu.

• Eat more slowly and concentrate on tasting and savoring your food. Put down your fork and breathe between bites. Talking to your table-mates is nice, too.

• Cut down on how many simple, refined carbohydrates you eat. These types of carbs are found mostly in white flour and white sugar foods like muffins, cookies, cake, breads, pasta, white rice, tortillas, and many cold breakfast cereals. These foods raise your blood sugar high and quickly. If you have type 2 diabetes, your body's response is to secrete a lot of insulin. Since insulin is a fat-storage hormone, it goes to work turning what calories you don't burn from these foods into fat. If you have type 1 diabetes, you'll need to take more insulin to cover these foods and the same scenario plays out.

• Leave something over on your plate. This is how I began cutting down on calories. I'd leave over a spoonful of mashed potatoes or a few bites of my turkey sandwich. It doesn't matter what it is, but you'll get in the habit of not cleaning your plate and eating less. Trust me, no children in China are going to go hungry because you're not cleaning your plate.

• Meet with a dietitian (ask your doctor for a referral) to create a meal plan. Your meal plan should keep your blood sugar, blood pressure, and cholesterol in check, and give you enough to eat to feel satisfied and lose some weight if you need to.

Tips to order a healthier meal in a restaurant:

• Take a look at the menu online at home and decide what you will order. You'll be less swayed by what your dining companions order.

• Ask the server not to bring bread to the table. If others want bread, return the bread basket to the server after they take what they want.

• When eating out, your hand makes a great guide for portion sizes: one cup is about the size of your fist. A half cup about the size of your open palm, a tablespoon about the size of your thumb, and a teaspoon the tip of your thumb.

• Share an appetizer and/or take part of your dinner home. My husband and I do this most times we eat out.

• Ask for sauces to be put on the side and only use a little.

• If your meal comes with a starchy food like potato or rice, and a non-starchy vegetable like broccoli or spinach, and you're beyond your daily carbohydrate limit, ask if they can hold the starch and double the green vegetable.

Do #2

Seek Health First from Your Foods

Before we had the many medicines we have today, physicians treated their patients with food and herbs. Granted, many of our modern pharmaceuticals can be, and are, life-saving, and I wouldn't want to get rid of them. Yet we seem to have forgotten the power of healthy foods to nourish us, prevent disease, and make and keep us well.

Try eating a healthy diet to improve your health before you ask your doctor for a pill. You may not need that pill. For better or for worse, the foods we eat affect our diabetes and the many conditions that often come with type 2 diabetes: obesity, high blood pressure, and high cholesterol.

People with diabetes are advised to follow the same general nutrition guidelines for health, (with an important note I'd like to add) that are recommended for all Americans: eat vegetables, fruits, whole grains, lean meats, poultry, fish, low-fat dairy, healthful fats, fiber, and occasional sweets—in sensible portions. Here's my note: 1) For people with diabetes, since grains and fruit will raise your blood sugar more significantly than the other foods (with the exception of sweets), consider eating less of them to help you keep your blood sugar in your target range more easily. I do, and it works for me. 2) Since some low-fat dairy foods contain artificial ingredients and/or more carbohydrates than their full-fat version, I read the labels and make my choice based on both the fat and carbohydrate content.

Ultimately, the best meal plan for you is the one that helps keep your blood sugar, cholesterol, blood pressure, and weight within your target range. And it should be one you can stick to. That means you can have occasional sweets and treats. And that's so much better than ripping someone's head off when what you really want is a bowl of ice cream.

Remember, what you put in your body every day builds the foundation of your health. Eating healthy foods has a curative and healing effect on our bodies, and our diabetes. Dr. Mark Hyman, author of *The Blood Sugar Solution*, says, "What you put on the end of a fork is more powerful than what you find in a bottle of pills." And unlike a bottle of pills, the only side effect of a healthy meal plan is a healthier you!

Quick-Starts

☐ **Always have some veggies and fruit washed and cut in your fridge.** This way they're easy to grab when you're hungry (instead of reaching for that giant-size bag of potato chips) and you can throw them in your bag when you're on the go.

☐ **Use the "Plate Method" to make a healthy meal:** Fill half your plate with low or non-starchy veggies like broccoli, asparagus, cauliflower, Brussels sprouts, string beans, mushrooms, peppers, or leafy greens; and some fruit. Fill one quarter with a whole grain like brown rice, barley, bulgur, or quinoa, or a starchy vegetable like corn or potatoes, or beans. Fill one quarter with protein like broiled, sauteed, roasted, or baked (not fried) fish; chicken or turkey without the skin; lean cuts of meat; tofu; or eggs.

Your Choice of More How-To's

☐ Instead of counting calories, choose foods that nourish your body. A meal of fat-free, sugar-free, refined processed foods is also nutrient-free.

Plus, it won't satisfy you for long compared to a meal of nutrient-dense whole foods like vegetables, lean meats, whole grains, and healthy fat.

☐ See if a supermarket near you uses the Nuval® nutritional scoring system. Nuval® scores food and beverages from 1 to 100 (1 being the least nutritious, 100 being the most nutritious). Choose items with the higher scores. Some of the markets that carry Nuval® scores are: Tops, King Kullen, Price Chopper, Hy-Vee, Lowe's, United Supermarkets, and Price Cuttter.

☐ Eat fruits and vegetables soon after you buy them, including those you put in the freezer. Over time, they lose some of their nutrients. Also, steam or microwave, rather than boil, your veggies to keep them vitamin rich.

☐ Take a cooking class to learn how to make tasty and healthy meals. It can be fun, and preparing and eating healthier meals at home will improve your overall health.

☐ Read magazines, articles on the internet, and books about what foods have a positive effect on blood sugar, blood pressure, cholesterol, and health.

☐ To ensure there's always something healthy in the house to eat, shop for fresh vegetables, fruits, meats, and poultry on the weekends and make nutritious stews, soups, and dishes you can freeze and serve during the week.

☐ Check labels for how much carbohydrate a food contains. Many processed foods like fruit yogurt and breakfast cereal may contain more carbs than you think because they have added sugar. While all carbohydrates break down in your body into glucose (sugar), the guideline for how much sugar you eat or drink, from the American Diabetes Association, is no more than six teaspoons (25 grams) a day for women and no more than nine teaspoons (37 grams) a day for men. Right now the average American consumes twenty-two teaspoons of sugar a day. Just one twelve ounce can of soda has 39 grams of sugar, more sugar than a man should get in a day!

☐ Add cinnamon to your cereal, yogurt, cottage cheese, and even spicy stews. While the verdict is inconclusive, some clinical trials have shown this fragrant spice to help lower blood sugar.

☐ Put more tumeric into your diet. Tumeric is a plant in the ginger family and has a peppery, warm fragrant flavor. It's what gives mustard its bright yellow color and is used in Indian curry dishes. In addition to having anti-inflammatory properties, tumeric has been found to improve beta (insulin-producing) cell function and reduce insulin-resistance in adults with pre-diabetes.

Healthy substitutions:

• You're better off eating fresh and frozen fruits and vegetables than chomping on vitamins and supplements. While a multi-vitamin may help cover your bases if your diet is lacking, know that vitamins and supplements don't give you the same health boost you get from the many, and perfect combination of, nutrients in whole foods. If your doctor prescribes a certain vitamin, follow doctor's orders. Otherwise, be aware that claims about the benefit of vitamins and supplements are mostly unproven, and some studies show certain vitamins and supplements create damage in our bodies.

• Cut down on sodas, soft drinks, and juices. If you drink three or more of these a day, start cutting down to no more than two. Then replace one of these with a glass of milk, which can help build bone density; or white or green teas, which have high levels of healthy anti-oxidants.

• Instead of bottled salad dressings, here's my everyday healthy dressing: a tablespoon or two of olive or flax oil, a splash of red wine vinegar or lemon, mustard for a little kick, and herbs like basil, oregano, rosemary, thyme. Here's a flavorful dressing recipe from nutrition-savvy Dr. Joel Fuhrman: combine about ½ cup of unsalted tomato sauce, 1 tablespoon raw creamy almond butter, and 1–2 tablespoons balsamic vinegar and mix. You can also add roasted garlic and sun dried tomatoes.

• Substitute almond meal for flour when baking to cut down on carbs. Almond meal has 5 grams of carb in ¼ cup, while white flour has 22 grams of carb, and buckwheat flour has 21 grams of carb, each per ¼ cup. A dietitian gave me this tip and says you can use almond meal in cupcakes, teacakes, bread, crackers, pie crust, and more by following the recipes on Elanaspantry.com. I now make my occasional whole grain pancakes and chocolate ginger biscotti with almond meal. And everyone's happy!

• Sugar substitutes like Equal, Sweet 'N Low and Splenda, and plant-based sweetener Stevia, have received cautious approval by the American Diabetes Association and the American Heart Association. However, many people who eat foods containing these types of sweeteners think they're saving so many calories that they actually end up rewarding themselves by eating foods that cause them to consume more calories in the long run. Also, many think, and I agree, that using a lot of these sweeteners keeps you craving sweets. Use these sweeteners, and eat foods with them, sparingly. Here's an utterly simple occasional treat I make with a sugar substitute: sprinkle Splenda or Stevia and cinnamon lightly on a piece of whole grain toast. If I put a few thin slices of apple or peach on the toast, I leave off the sweetener.

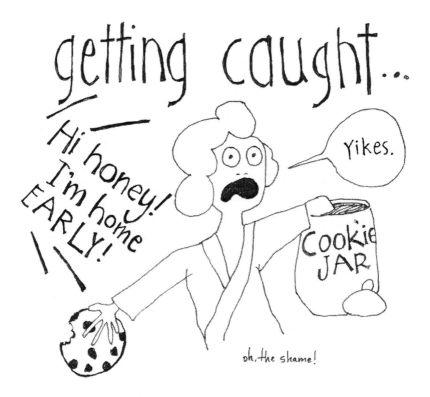

Do #3

Make Your Kitchen a Shrine to Heart Health

Two out of three people with type 2 diabetes will die of a heart attack or stroke, and many already have some heart disease when diagnosed. So the more heart-healthy foods you eat, the less likely you'll be the one in the ambulance racing to the ER with a heart attack.

Heart-healthy foods include vegetables and fruit; legumes (foods like peas, beans, lentils, and peanuts); raw unsalted nuts; and low-fat dairy, chicken and fish. Overall, these foods supply nutrients that protect your heart. Even if your arteries already have some fatty build-up, a heart-healthy diet may slow its progress. The American Heart Association says a heart-healthy diet can also lower blood pressure, cholesterol, and weight, all of which reduce the risk of heart disease.

Many of these heart-healthy foods also supply valuable fiber. Fiber helps lower cholesterol, aids your digestive process, promotes weight loss, and reduces inflammation. Inflammation may contribute to causing heart problems as well as some cancers. The USDA recommends 14 grams of fiber for every 1,000 calories you eat in a day. The recommendation is for women to eat around 1,600–2,200 calories a day, and for men around 2,400–3,000 calories, depending on age and activity. That's about 20 to 35 grams of fiber for most people. And most people don't get nearly that much. The one fruit you eat a day only supplies between 2 and 7 grams of fiber, and a slice of ordinary bread has only 2 grams.

So when you make out your shopping list be sure to include these heart-healthy winners: salmon, olive oil, oats, apples, almonds, walnuts, pistachios, 100 percent whole grains, green leafy vegetables, tomatoes, and soy. Then toss the Cheese Doodles—or at least stash them in the back of the cupboard where, maybe, you'll find them in a few years by accident and they'll be too gross to eat!

Also, a glass of red wine a day is not only good for the spirit, but also your heart. It contains resveratrol, an anti-oxidant that's thought to help prevent heart disease by protecting your body against artery damage. Don't start drinking if you don't already, but if you do, the recommendation is one glass a day for women and no more than two for men.

Quick-Starts

☐ **Eat 3.5 ounces of fish at least twice a week.** Eat it baked, sautéed, or grilled, not fried. Fish is low in saturated fat and a good source of protein and heart-healthy omega-3 fatty acids. The American Heart Association says omega-3 fatty acids decrease your risk of arrhythmias (abnormal heartbeats that can lead to sudden death), lower triglyceride levels, slightly lower blood pressure, and slow the growth of plaque in your arteries. Fatty fish like salmon, mackerel, herring, lake trout, sardines, and albacore tuna are high in omega-3 fatty acids.

☐ **Trim the fat off red meats.** All meat will have some white lines of fat running through it that keep the meat tender. That's fine. But cut away any thick chunks of pure white fat. Most think this is unhealthy and it adds extra calories.

Your Choice of More How-To's

☐ Enjoy your eggs, they're great protein. Many experts say cholesterol in food does not raise our cholesterol, and I agree. However, if you think differently, you can always make two or three eggs and throw away one or two of the yolks.

☐ When dining out, if the restaurant offers them, choose "heart-healthy" menu items. If you see "low-fat" items on the menu, ask the server if they contain sugar. If so, ask how much. Many times sugar goes into a dish when fat comes out. My go-to meal, especially since I travel a lot, is broiled salmon and a green vegetable.

☐ Get more fiber in your diet. If you're not used to eating fiber, increase your intake slowly. Eating too much fiber too quickly can upset your stomach and make you bloated and gassy. Adding an apple a day is a good way to start. Then add some non-starchy veggies like broccoli, cauliflower, or spinach to your meals. Then add any kind of bean, lentils, cooked peas, brown rice, edamame, and grains like barley and steel cut oatmeal.

☐ If you love crispy chicken skin, a bit now and then won't hurt you. A twelve-ounce chicken breast, which is four times the recommended serving of three ounces (the size of your palm), with the skin contains just 2.5 grams of saturated fat and fifty calories more than without the skin. Remember, for a serving, divide that by four.

☐ Stay away from fried foods—far, far away! Prepare lean meats and poultry by broiling, baking, grilling, or sautéing.

☐ If you don't eat two meals of fatty fish a week, discuss with your doctor or a dietitian whether adding a fish oil supplement to your meal plan would be a good idea.

Do #4

Toss a Rainbow on Your Plate

No, this doesn't require a rainstorm or a crane. Rather, it's about eating a variety of colorful vegetables and fruits each day. Dietary experts recommend five to nine servings of vegetables and fruit a day to get essential vitamins, minerals, and some powerhouse nutrients into our meal plans. The colorful skin—and insides—of veggies and fruits are loaded with disease-fighting substances that help reduce tissue damage, prevent certain cancers, enhance our immune system, and reduce the risk for chronic diseases.

If you like to measure, the United States Department of Agriculture (USDA) charts the recommendation as at least two and a half cups of vegetables and two cups of fruit each day. The USDA defines a serving size for fruit and veggies as a half-cup, except for whole fruits like an apple or orange, which count as one serving each. Low-cal greens, like spinach and lettuce, get a larger serving size, one cup. Since individual needs vary—and fruit will raise your blood sugar—how much fruit you eat should also depend on your age, gender, and physical activity.

If you don't eat a lot of vegetables, you have a whole new world to discover. There are flower bud, and simple bud, vegetables like broccoli, cauliflower, artichokes, and Brussels sprouts. These are low in carbs, full of vitamins and minerals, and help to reduce inflammation. There are leafy vegetables like kale, collard greens, spinach, arugula, bok choy, chard, and others. Kale has become a superstar among veggies. It has almost no carbs, is high in fiber, contains minerals that are hard to get from other foods, and it scores off the chart for anti-inflammatory properties. Sweet corn, peas, and beans are considered seed vegetables. These are a bit higher in carbs. Rounding out the list are stem vegetables like celery and rhubarb; shoots like asparagus; sprouts like soybeans and alfalfa; roots like carrots, beets, and radishes; bulbs like onions and garlic; and tubers like potatoes. Whew! All these veggies vary in how many carbohydrates, vitamins, and minerals they contain. By combining them, you'll cover the bases for essential nutrients and keep yourself from getting bored.

As for fruit, eating it may protect you against diabetic retinopathy (eye disease). A study conducted in Japan showed people who ate nine ounces of fruit a day (an apple is about six ounces) had half the chance of developing retinopathy. While the study didn't show cause and effect, it did show a link.

All said, to get the maximum amount of nutrients and a lower rise in your blood sugar, you're best off to favor veggies over fruit, but by all means include both. And mix up the colors. Steam red peppers, orange carrots, yellow onions, purple eggplant, green broccoli, and white cauliflower for your veggies for dinner. Follow with a small fruit salad of red strawberries, orange apricots, yellow peaches, blueberries—well, you get the idea, just think rainbow.

Quick-Starts

☐ **Fold assorted veggies into an omelet** like peppers, mushrooms, asparagus, tomatoes and onions. Put broccoli, peas, and carrots in a whole wheat pasta dish or in a low-sodium (salt) vegetable-based soup. Top your breakfast cereal with blueberries and peaches, and munch on raw carrots, celery, squash, broccoli, and asparagus with a lower-fat dip like hummus.

☐ **Eat frozen fruits and vegetables when fresh aren't available.** They may be even tastier, and cheaper.

Your Choice of More How-To's

☐ Pick up nutrition advocate, Dr. Neal Barnard, and nutritionist Robyn Webb's book, *The Get Healthy, Go Vegan Cookbook*. It has healthy vegan recipes and tips for people who want to lose weight, cut cholesterol, and reverse the symptoms of type 2 diabetes.

☐ To preserve veggies' nutrients and flavor, steam or sauté them with a little olive oil, bake or roast them with herbs, and toss the ones you can eat raw in salads.

☐ Substitute a portabella mushroom for the bun on your veggie burger.

☐ For a quick snack, put veggies into the microwave for two minutes. I microwave my Brussels sprouts and love the chewy, crunchy texture.

☐ Put bananas and unripe strawberries with some Splenda on them into the freezer. When you take them out and let them defrost, they're sweet and delicious.

☐ While it doesn't have the fiber benefit of whole vegetables, fresh vegetable juice, or a can of low-sodium V8, is an easy way to get extra servings of vegetables.

☐ For fresh fruit salad, stick to one portion size (three heaping tablespoons). As healthful as fruit is, most are high in carbohydrates and all raise your blood sugar. Fruits that typically raise your blood sugar less include berries, cherries, apples, pears, grapefruit, plums, and peaches. A higher blood sugar rise will come from pineapple, raisins, mangoes, papaya, watermelon, and any canned fruit that comes in sweet syrup.

☐ Check this website for fruit and veggie portion sizes: nhs.uk/Livewell/ 5ADAY/Documents/Downloads/5ADAY_portion_guide.pdf.

Do #5

Get "the Skinny" on Fat

There's much debate about what makes us fat, other than eating more calories than we burn. And in an effort to get Americans to lose weight, we've been told to give up fat. Yet, Americans are fatter than ever.

It's true one gram of fat contains more calories than protein or carbohydrate. A gram of fat has nine calories, compared to four calories in a gram of protein and carbohydrate. But many scientists and dietitians are changing their opinions about fat's effect on making us fat. After all, as a nation that gave up fat for carbohydrates a decade ago, we've only gotten fatter. Studies now show that carbohydrates we eat and don't burn get stored in the body as fat—and that may be more responsible for making us fat!

Here's how it works: you eat sugary and starchy foods (carbohydrates) and they break down into sugar in your bloodstream. If your body still produces insulin, your body releases and circulates more insulin to bring your blood sugar back to normal. If you have type 1 diabetes, you take extra insulin to cover these foods and you have more insulin circulating in your blood stream. But insulin is also a fat storage hormone, so the excess sugar that you don't burn as energy gets stored as fat on your belly, hips, buttocks, and thighs.

Carbohydrate foods also tend to raise our appetite so we tend to eat more, while fats satisfy our appetite so we tend to eat less. Some evidence also suggests that following a diet higher in healthy fat and lower in carbohydrates may help with blood sugar control. In a recent study, people with type 2 diabetes were divided into two groups. One followed a low-carbohydrate/higher-fat diet, and the other a low-fat/ higher carbohydrate diet. People in both groups lost about nine pounds, but people who ate the lower-carb/higher fat diet saw their HbA1c (a measure of average blood sugar over the past two to three months) drop from 7.5% to 7% and their insulin dose drop 30 percent! Plus, their HDL (healthy cholesterol) went up.

Will eating too much fat make you fat? Sure. But don't cut fat out of your diet. Eat fewer unhealthy fats and more healthy fats. (See Do #6. Keep Your Body Glowing with "Good" Fats.) In the end you'll feel fuller, be satisfied with fewer calories, and perhaps need less medicine.

Quick-Starts

☐ **This week eat half the amount of an unhealthy fat you eat** like packaged snack foods, fried dishes, commercially-baked cookies, cakes, doughnuts, or muffins.

☐ **Have the full-fat version of a food if the low-fat version has more carbohydrates.** For example, Kraft Thousand Island dressing has 5 carbs, yet Wishbone Fat Free Thousand Island dressing has 9.

Your Choice of More How-To's

☐ If your meal plan calls for 45 to 60 grams of carbohydrates per meal and you're struggling to lose weight, ask your health care provider whether it wouldn't be better to reduce the carbs and add healthy fats and a little more protein.

☐ Pour two tablespoons of water into a shot glass and mark the line with a marker. Now you have an easy measure for salad dressing.

☐ Skip the bagel and low-fat cream cheese for breakfast and instead eat a bowl of steel cut oatmeal. Check out my own recipe under "Do #11. Turn Ho-Hum Oatmeal into Your 'Can't-Wait-For' Breakfast."

☐ To know roughly how many calories you should eat in a day to lose some weight, first figure out how many pounds you would weigh if you lost 7 percent of your body weight. For instance, if you weigh 200 pounds now and lose 7 percent of your body weight, you will weigh 186 pounds. Then create a meal plan in which you eat the daily number of calories to sustain a weight of 186 pounds. Here's an easy formula: If you're not active, 186 pounds x 10 calories/pound = 1,860 calories/day. If you are active, 186 pounds x 12–13 calories/pound = 2,232–2,418 calories/day.

Do #6

Keep Your Body Glowing with "Good" Fats

Fat has gotten a bad rap, but healthy, unsaturated fats are good for you. So load the pantry with unsalted nuts; seeds; avocados; legumes; olives; oils like extra virgin olive, flax, and coconut; as well as peanut and grapeseed oil, which cook better on high heat. The United States Department of Agriculture (USDA) recommends that a third of our daily calories come from healthy fats in foods like these.

Healthy fats help us absorb all the healthy stuff—vitamins, minerals, and antioxidants—in other foods. They supply energy, help our bodies build cell membranes; keep a sparkle in our eyes; add a shine to our skin and hair; and strengthen our digestive, nervous and immune systems. And all of these systems are more vulnerable when you have diabetes.

Studies have also shown that good fats reduce the risk of heart disease, certain cancers, obesity, arthritis, Alzheimer's, depression, joint pain, and inflammation. Step right up and eat your fats!

Omega-3 fatty acids are a particularly healthy fat that most people don't get enough of. They help control blood clotting, lower blood pressure, lower LDL (lousy) cholesterol and triglycerides, and raise HDL (healthy) cholesterol. They also decrease the growth of plaque that can create blockages in an artery and may lead to a stroke or a heart attack.

Some omega-3 stars include fatty fish such as salmon, herring, mackerel, anchovies, and sardines; ground flax seeds; flax seed oil; and walnuts. I add ground flax seeds and sometimes walnuts to my morning cereal and love the crunch and texture.

As for saturated fat (the fat in animal foods like steak and eggs), most dietitians say stay away, yet some experts side with a moderate intake. Since there really is no definitive answer yet whether saturated fat is bad for us, and our overall health doesn't depend on any one thing you eat or don't eat, my mantra is moderation: enjoy these foods occasionally, not every day.

There is, however, a type of fat that everyone agrees is bad for you: trans fats. If you've formed a little love-in with trans fats, it's time to stop. Trans fats also appear on a label as "hydrogenated" or "partially hydrogenated oil." Trans fats are added to foods to lengthen *their* life—not yours. These unhealthy fats raise LDL (lousy) cholesterol and lower HDL (healthy) cholesterol, boo! Unfortunately, you'll find them lurking in most baked goods like cookies, crackers, cakes and muffins, pizza dough, fried foods like doughnuts, French fries, chicken nuggets, taco shells, potato and corn chips, solid fats like stick margarine, and pre-mixed products like cake and pancake mix. My advice: If you just can't throw them out, don't restock them when you run out.

Quick-Starts

☐ **Keep your pantry free of products that list "hydrogenated" or "partially hydrogenated oil" in the ingredients.** Even if a food claims to be trans-fat-free, the word "hydrogenated" in the ingredient list tells you that it isn't.

☐ **At least twice a week replace processed meats like bacon, hot dogs, cold cuts, spareribs, and sausage with fresh or canned tuna or salmon.** Processed meats are high in fat and sodium (salt) and linked to certain cancers. *Consumer Reports* says light tuna has less mercury than white tuna.

Your Choice of More How-To's

☐ Choose white meats, like chicken and turkey, and pork, more often than red meats. When you do eat red meat, choose lean cuts, and if you go to a butcher have him trim off the fat.

☐ Eat fewer fried foods, biscuits, and other baked goods, and eat them less often.

☐ Have what my husband eats for breakfast: two pieces of fruit, usually an apple and small banana and a small handful of walnuts, almonds, and macadamia nuts. He switched to this breakfast when a heart surgeon friend of ours told us how our blood gets "dirty" when we eat poor quality fats.

☐ Sprinkle a few nuts of any variety and sunflower seeds on your cereal, salad, and veggies.

☐ Use thin slices of avocado as a sandwich spread instead of commercial spreads.

☐ Use 1 to 2 tablespoons of extra virgin olive oil, flaxseed oil, coconut oil, sesame oil, or peanut oil, as well as lemon, balsamic or red wine vinegar, mustard, and herbs as a salad dressing instead of a creamy bottled dressing.

Do #7

Shun "Made for Diabetics" Foods

If marketers could sell grass to cows, they'd find a way. No one needs to eat "made for diabetics" foods. These foods often contain more carbohydrates or fat than the real foods they're replacing. Let's face it, the people who benefit the most from these products are mostly the manufacturers who charge extra high prices.

Take a look: Chips Ahoy Chocolate Chip cookies contain 5.2 grams of fat while Murray Sugar-Free Chocolate Chip cookies contain 6 grams of fat. Kellogg's Special K cereal, which is marketed to help decrease your waistline, has twenty calories more than Kellogg's Corn Flakes. It also has .5 grams of fat, while Kellogg's Corn Flakes has no fat. Comparing sugar-free Reese's Peanut Butter Cups to the regular version, the sugar-free product has the same amount of fat and 1 less carbohydrate, but it contains the sugar alcohol maltitol, which in small quantities may be okay but is not recommended in larger quantities.

Many sugar-free sweets contain sugar alcohols. In addition to maltitol, they come with names like xylitol, isomalt, sorbitol, lactitol and mannitol. Because your body doesn't completely absorb sugar alcohols, they provide fewer calories and have less impact on your blood sugar. But they can also ferment in your intestines and cause uncomfortable bloating, gas, or diarrhea. If you have this reaction to a sugar-free food, check for sugar alcohols on the label.

Quick-Starts

☐ **Have one serving of a delicious fruit: three fresh figs, a juicy ripe peach, one cup of ripe strawberries, a small banana, or three pineapple slices** instead of a serving of a sweet that says "Made for Diabetics."

☐ **If you have a specific craving, like "I NEED CHOCOLATE OR I'LL HURT YOU!!!"** have one or two small squares of a premium chocolate and savor it. Feel it melt on your tongue and enjoy the heck out of it. By the way, the darker the chocolate, the more healthy antioxidants it contains. Personally, I'm an 85% Extra Dark Lindt chocolate fan.

Your Choice of More How-To's

☐ Eat the real thing and eat one portion. Put a serving in a bowl and put the rest away.

☐ Cut down on your use of artificial sweeteners. The jury is still out as to whether or not they are truly safe and many think they keep us craving sweets.

☐ If you feel the need to finish a box of candy, cookies, or salty snack foods once you start, buy them in small, single serving 100 calorie packages. While I don't recommend eating many of these because they are mostly empty calories and high in unhealthy fat, at least this way you can enjoy an occasional sweet or salty snack and have built-in portion control. Oreos, Chips Ahoy, Lorna Doone, Doritos, Ritz crackers, and other snack foods come packaged this way.

☐ If you like a "made for diabetic" or "no-sugar" food and it contains fewer carbohydrates and less fat than the real thing, and not a long list of artificial ingredients, enjoy it. Some fruit preserves fill the bill.

☐ For chocolate, check out the Charles Bar at charlesbarcandy.com, created by celebrity chef and diabetes advocate, Charles Mattocks. It's premium Belgian chocolate and diabetic-friendly: sugar-free, gluten-free, and low in carbs.

Do #8

Have Less Maybe "Scary Dairy"

I call it "scary dairy" because dairy foods contain roughly 50 to 60 percent saturated fat and the American Heart Association links saturated fat to heart disease. And people with type 2 diabetes are three times more likely to suffer from heart disease. The American Heart Association recommends most people limit their saturated fat to fewer than 16 grams a day. In terms of dairy, that looks like a mere two tablespoons of butter.

The United States Department of Agriculture (USDA) gives the guideline for dairy as three cups of dairy a day. What does this look like? A glass of milk, pat of butter, and ½ cup of cottage cheese; or a glass of milk, 1.5 ounces of cheese (think two Domino pieces), and ½ cup of ice cream (think half the size of a baseball); or one and a half scoops of a premium ice cream, like Ben and Jerry's or Haagen-Daz.

While most nutritionists stress low-fat dairy over full-fat dairy, sometimes you're trading fat for more carbohydrates or artificial ingredients. Recent research also says there's no real evidence that saturated fat from dairy causes more risk for heart disease. Plus, often when people eat low-fat foods, their hunger drives them to eat more calories than they would have eating the regular versions.

Here's my policy: I eat dairy foods on a spectrum—non-fat cottage cheese, 2% Greek yogurt, lower- and full-fat cheeses, and yes, half and half in my coffee. So while the verdict is still out on this one, what most doctors and dietitians agree on, is that we shouldn't be eating *a lot of* saturated fat.

These dairy foods have a high saturated fat content:

- Butter

- Cheese

- Cream cheese

- Some yogurts

- Sour cream

- Whipped cream

- Whole milk

Since dairy supplies much-needed calcium to build strong bones, many nutritionists and doctors, like diabetes specialist Dr. Neal Barnard, recommend getting your calcium from eating more dark, green leafy vegetables and beans if you choose to cut down on dairy.

I must also mention that some nutritionists and medical professionals say we shouldn't eat dairy at all. Integrative medicine authority and author of *The Blood Sugar Solution*, Dr. Mark Hyman, says that proteins found in dairy foods can create insulin imbalances. According to Dr. Hyman, drinking a glass of milk can spike insulin levels (provided you're still making insulin) 300 percent and contribute to obesity and pre-diabetes.

Quick-Starts

☐ **Use lower-fat dairy products when they don't contain artificial ingredients or many more carbs than their full-fat version.**

☐ **Eat half your usual amount of New York cheesecake.** *Sigh,* I know, but your body will thank you.

Your Choice of More How-To's

☐ Read the label and use your common sense. If a lower fat food has one or two more carbohydrates, but a lot less fat and calories and you're watching your weight, no reason not to use it. But look at this example: 1 cup of full-fat yogurt has 138 calories, 7 grams of fat and 11 grams of carbohydrate. The non-fat version has 127 calories, 0.4 grams of fat, and 17 grams of carb. The calorie savings is small, but the carb increase is not—and carbohydrates you don't burn get stored as fat. Here I'd eat the full-fat yogurt.

☐ These substitutions will let you lower the amount of dairy fat you eat without increasing the carbs. Choose skim, 1%, or 2% milk instead of whole milk. All contain roughly 11.5 grams of carbs per cup. Unsweetened almond and soy milks are another alternative for full fat milk. Almond milk contains only 2–4 grams of carbs per cup and soy milk only 4 grams of carbs per cup. Alert: rice milk contains 23 grams of carbs per cup.

☐ Switch to Greek yogurt. It has about twice the protein of regular yogurt, and fewer carbohydrates.

☐ Substitute whipped butter for stick butter. It's lower in saturated fat and calories. Breakstone's and Land O' Lakes both make good whipped butters.

☐ If you like cheese, include lower fat cheeses in your meal plan like Jarlsberg or feta. Eat full-fat cheese, like brie, gruyere, and blue cheese, occasionally and in small amounts.

☐ When using cheese to flavor a dish or sauce pick a mature, strong-flavored cheese. These will give you more flavor than young or mild-tasting cheeses, so you can use less.

Do #9

Rethink Your Love Affair with Salt

Someone once said to me, "Why do we salt our food before we even taste it?" It made me think, so I stopped salting my food. After two weeks, if I tasted something salty, it was soooo salty.

It's not really salt that's the problem when we hear Americans should eat less salt, it's sodium. Sodium makes up 40 percent of salt, and while it's essential for regulating our body's fluids and blood pressure, too much sodium raises blood pressure and, you guessed it: people with diabetes are at greater risk for high blood pressure. Plus, high blood pressure can contribute to heart disease, which you may already know people with diabetes are at higher risk for.

Here's what you may not know: the United States Department of Agriculture (USDA) Dietary Guideline recommends we get no more than 2,300 mg of sodium per day—that's a teaspoon of salt. If you are over 51, African American, or have high blood pressure, chronic kidney disease, or diabetes, the recommendation is 1,500 milligrams of sodium per day—that's about two-thirds of a teaspoon.

Most Americans consume more than 3,400 mg of sodium each day. It's not so hard to understand once you discover that 80 percent of our sodium comes from restaurant and processed foods like frozen pizza and other frozen entrees, hot dogs, fresh meats, condiments, canned soups, and snack foods. A rack of baby back ribs has 20,000 mg of sodium— that's 10 teaspoons! Meanwhile that little salt shaker on the table? It only supplies about 6 percent of the sodium in your diet.

Quick-Starts

☐ **Check the sodium (salt) amount on any packaged food you consume**. No one product should have more than 500 mg of sodium per serving.

☐ **Choose unsalted nuts, pretzels, and crackers** over salted nuts, pretzels, and crackers.

Your Choice of More How-To's

☐ Cut out or cut down on the cured meats you eat such as bacon and sausage, lunch meat, packaged or prepared foods, and snack foods like salted pretzels and chips. These foods are high in sodium.

☐ Use high sodium salad dressing and condiments sparingly. These include canned and pickled vegetables, pickles, olives, and ketchup. Or choose low-sodium versions.

☐ When you eat out ask if the chef will prepare the dish with no or less salt.

☐ Ask for sauces on the side and use just a little. Most sauces are high in sodium. The occasional times I order ribs, I order them dry if I can. If not, I scrape the sauce off when they come to the table.

☐ Check out the DASH eating plan at dashdiet.org. It's a balanced eating plan to promote heart health that's low in sodium and emphasizes vegetables and fruit, lean protein, and whole grains.

☐ Instead of salt, use herbs like rosemary, thyme, basil, and oregano, and/or lemon or vinegar in your cooking. Also, choose low-salt stock cubes if making soups.

☐ If you have high blood pressure, choose foods that say "low sodium" (140 mg or less salt per serving) or "no salt added." If you just want to cut back, choose "reduced sodium" products. They usually have 25 percent less salt.

☐ Ask your doctor or dietitian to recommend a salt substitute. This is especially important if you're on a diuretic or water pill.

Do #10

Fall Madly in Love with Complex Carbs

You may have heard people call carbohydrates "bad" and "good." What those labels commonly refer to are foods that contain simple carbohydrates ("bad") and complex carbohydrates ("good"). Now it gets even trickier. For simplicity's sake, I'm going to divide simple carbohydrates into three categories. The first are foods that contain natural sugars within them: mostly fruits, milk, and milk products. The second are foods to which sugar has been added, like cake, candy, cookies, muffins, scones, cupcakes, soda, fruit juice, syrups, chips, cold breakfast cereals, and most supermarket breads. The third are foods that act like simple carbohydrates in the body, like white potatoes, white rice, white bread, and white pasta.

While fruits and vegetables naturally contain sugar, their high fiber content, vitamins, and minerals makes them quite nutritious. Foods that have added sugar, however, are low in fiber and provide lots of calories with little, if any, nutrition. Also, I can attest to the fact that eating too many potato chips and shortbread cookies washed down with sweet tea (well it was ages ago!) can lead to feeling pretty crummy, along with mood swings, fatigue, cravings, and not thinking very clearly. I'll get to the "white" foods in a minute.

Simple carbohydrates are quick for your body to digest. They also raise your blood sugar quickly and higher than other foods do. In response, if you're still making insulin, your body will release a surge of insulin. If you're not making insulin, you may take extra insulin to cover your blood sugar rise. Lots of insulin circulating in your bloodstream can drop your blood sugar too low and it can also contribute to weight gain. Simple carbohydrates with added sugar are also like a siren to your taste buds, "More, more…please, eat more," they call. And the cycle starts again with the next meal or snack.

Complex carbohydrates, on the other hand, contain starch and fiber. For this reason, they take longer to break down into glucose (sugar in your blood) and so they raise your blood sugar more slowly and evenly than simple carbohydrates. They actually help you maintain more energy and more stable blood sugars. Complex carbs are powerhouse foods like 100% whole, intact grains—barley, whole oats, popcorn, bulgur, millet, quinoa, and buckwheat. These grains still have their nutrient-dense outer layer of bran and germ.

Now back to our "white" foods. When eating them in their "brown" state—sweet potatoes, brown rice, whole grain bread, and whole wheat pasta—they act as complex carbs in your body. Other complex carbs include: beans, lentils, nuts, and seeds; vegetables like sweet potato, winter squash, beets, peas, corn, and carrots for their starch content; low-starch, but high-fiber vegetables like broccoli, kale, Brussels sprouts, cauliflower, green beans, asparagus, peppers, zucchini, artichoke, eggplant, spinach, okra, pea pods, snap peas, mushrooms, onions, cabbage, celery, cucumber, all types of lettuces and sprouts.

Unlike simple carbs, complex carbohydrates are rich in vitamins, minerals, and health-promoting nutrients. They promote clear thinking, keep your mood more stable, and can help you lose weight because they keep you full longer and don't spike your blood sugar or your appetite. The simple rule of thumb is you're better off eating more complex carbohydrates than simple. My favorite complex carb is a sweet and nutty-tasting baked sweet potato with nothing on it. It's delicious hot or cold.

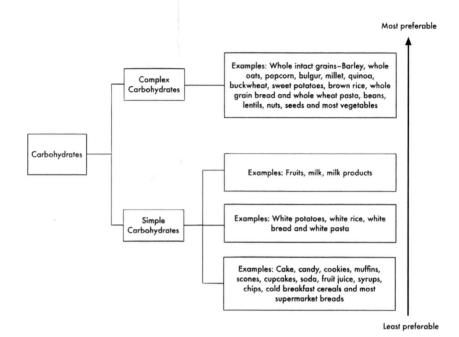

Diagram 1: Simple and complex carbohydrates

Now that you know all this, what you also need to know is different people's digestive systems handle different carbohydrates a little differently. Each of us breaks down the same carbohydrates and absorbs them at different rates, in part depending upon what else we're eating with them. So, while these guidelines are generally true, you need to see how these foods affect your blood sugar.

In the past decade, two ranking systems have emerged for carbohydrate foods. They're called the Glycemic Index (GI) and Glycemic Load (GL). Both offer a guide to how carbohydrate foods impact blood sugar. The lower the ranking of a food, the less impact on blood sugar. The Glycemic Load goes one step further than the Glycemic Index by taking into consideration a typical serving size of each food. GL values are considered more precise since they're based on the amount of food you normally eat, but both are good to become familiar with.

Quick-Starts

☐ **Add beans to your meals.** These complex carbs are winners for filling you up and keeping your blood sugar stable. Choose from any bean: black, kidney, pinto, white, navy, chickpeas, and lentils. Toss them into soups, salads, and pasta dishes. Just half a cup of canned chickpeas in tonight's salad will add 6 grams of fiber and 6 grams of protein. One cup of beans (⅓ – ½ cup is a serving) is loaded with protein, has only 1 gram of fat and 15 grams of fiber. *Tip: You can use canned or dried beans. For canned beans, discard the water and rinse them well before using to get rid of excess salt. Soak dried beans overnight, discard the water the next morning, and cook them in fresh water. You'll cut down on the gas beans can produce.*

☐ **Eat lower GI foods at breakfast** like eggs; Greek yogurt; tofu; oatmeal; 100 percent whole grains; fruits like grapefruit, prunes, and cherries; nuts and seeds; barley; and flax seed. Avoid muffins, danish, scones, and Pop Tarts. Research shows starting the day with a lower GI breakfast may prevent a spike in your blood sugar throughout the morning, up to and after lunch.

Your Choice of More How-To's

☐ Add more vegetables, fiber, and protein to your diet to slow the rise in your blood sugar. If you have type 2 diabetes, the insulin you produce may be enough to cover the slower rise in blood sugar from these foods.

☐ Eat fruit instead of drinking fruit juice. Fruit has healthy fiber and will also raise your blood sugar more slowly than juice. If you do drink fruit juice, pour half a glass of juice and fill the rest of the glass with seltzer or club soda. It's actually quite refreshing.

☐ Choose water instead of sugary sodas. Add a slice of lemon for some zest.

☐ Make slow-cooking steel cut oatmeal on the weekends. You can freeze batches and defrost them for use during the week. (See "Do #11. Turn Ho-Hum Oatmeal into Your 'Can't-Wait-For' Breakfast.")

☐ Choose breakfast cereals that don't contain added sugars.

☐ Buy breads that list "whole grains" as the first ingredient and ones where you can actually see the grains. You'll find these in health food stores if your local supermarket doesn't carry them. Avoid breads that list "enriched wheat flour" as the first ingredient. These breads have lost eleven vitamins and minerals in the flour processing. Breads that say "enriched" also contain added sugar and/or fat.

☐ Substitute barley for white rice. For many people it doesn't raise blood sugar as much, and it's a tasty addition to soups, stews, and salads.

These ingredients in a food are added sugars:

Brown sugar, corn sweetener, corn syrup, dextrose, fructose, fruit juice concentrates, glucose, high-fructose corn syrup, honey, invert sugar, lactose, maltose, malt syrup, molasses, raw sugar, sucrose, sugar, and syrup. The closer to the top of the list, the more of that sugar is in the food.

Glycemic Index and Glycemic Load:

• Get a book that lists the Glycemic Index and Glycemic Load of foods. You can also view a list online at: http://www.health.harvard.edu/newsweek/Glycemic_index_and_glycemic_load_for_100_foods.htm.

• Rule of thumb: Eat more foods with a low GL (under 10). These tend to be high-fiber vegetables and fruit, legumes, beans, and bran cereals. Eat fewer foods with a high GL (over 20), like candy, most baked goods made with white flour, and most cold breakfast cereals.

• Substitute lower GI and GL foods in place of higher GI and GL foods. For instance, substitute a bean casserole for pasta, sweet potatoes for white potatoes, sprouted grain, pumpernickel, and rye bread for white and whole wheat bread. When I make pasta at home, I use Dreamfields Pasta. Its Glycemic Index is 13, while other pastas typically have a GI of 38.

• Be aware the same foods can have a different GI and GL, depending on how they are prepared. For instance, microwaving a potato or beet raises their GI and GL because much of their carbohydrate converts into glucose. However, cooking pasta al dente (boiled for 8 minutes) gives it a lower GI and GL than cooking it until it's soft (boiled for 20 minutes).

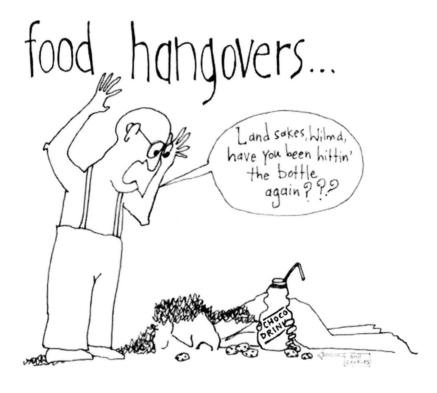

Do #11

Turn Ho-Hum Oatmeal into Your "Can't-Wait-For" Breakfast

Very often when I talk to fellow people with diabetes, I'm asked, "What do you eat for breakfast?" I almost always start the day with steel cut oatmeal and I'm going to share my special recipe with you. Steel cut oatmeal is one of the healthiest breakfasts you can eat. Preparing it the way I do, I find it so delicious, it's easy for me to forget how healthy oatmeal is. If you follow this recipe, you'll enjoy a breakfast cereal that's chewy, grainy, and nutty; cool and creamy; and much healthier than most highly processed cold breakfast cereals.

Besides satisfying your taste buds, oatmeal is a complex carbohydrate like we talked about in "Do #10. Fall Madly in Love with Complex Carbs." Oatmeal packs a nutritional punch: its 4 grams of heart-healthy soluble and insoluble fiber helps lower LDL (lousy) cholesterol and blood pressure. It's also a powerhouse of nutrients including vitamin E, zinc, selenium, copper, iron, manganese, magnesium, and cancer-fighting antioxidants.

I recommend steel cut oatmeal, over rolled oats, because it digests more slowly, helping you to avoid blood sugar spikes. But if you don't have time to make the steel cut version, rolled oats is a healthier choice than most cold breakfast cereals. Oatmeal has no additives and just over half the amount of carbohydrates as found in many cold cereals. Plus you won't need to add any sweetener or flavoring to this delish dish.

Quick-Starts

☐ **This week grab a can of steel cut oatmeal off the shelf of a nearby supermarket,** Trader Joe's, Whole Foods, or health food store.

☐ **Make a big batch of steel cut oatmeal on the weekends and freeze in single servings** you can defrost throughout the week.

Your Choice More of How-To's

☐ You can make steel cut oatmeal overnight in a two-quart crock pot so it's ready the next morning. Spray a little cooking spray in your crockpot to prevent the oatmeal from sticking. Then place 1 cup steel cut oats, 4 cups of water, ½ cup milk, ¼ cup brown sugar (optional), ½ teaspoon salt, 1 tablespoon butter (optional), ½ teaspoon vanilla extract, and 1 teaspoon cinnamon. You can also add ⅓ cup dried fruit like raisins, apricots, or prunes, or ½ cup fresh apple slices. Combine, cover, and cook on low for six to eight hours while you snooze. When you wake up, your house will smell warm and toasty AND breakfast will be made! Serve with some milk and nuts.

☐ Here's my own personal oatmeal recipe. My best guess is a single serving has about 34 carbs.

○ Place in a small bowl you love, 1 teaspoon raw sunflower seeds and 2 tablespoons ground flaxseeds. (Start with 1 teaspoon of flaxseeds at first and work up slowly, since they can irritate your stomach or cause diarrhea if you're not used to them.)

○ Cook ⅔ of a serving of steel-cut oatmeal. I use Country Choice Organic Irish Style Steel Cut Oats, which you can find at Trader Joe's. Many people like equally good McCann's Steel Cut Oatmeal. Add to dry ingredients and mix.

○ Top with your choice of fruit: a small handful of berries and a few bite-sized Granny Smith apple pieces or ⅓ of a cup of peach, pear, apricot or fig; 1 heaping tablespoon non-fat cottage cheese; 1 heaping tablespoon 2% Greek yogurt; 1 level tablespoon creamy or crunchy natural peanut butter; 1 level tablespoon raw natural almond butter; and cinnamon (optional).

○ Eat, sigh, savor, and know you did a good thing for your body!

☐ When traveling, I take with me individual envelopes of unflavored instant oatmeal and nuts. There's almost always a water cooker or coffee maker in a hotel room to make a nutritious mug of oatmeal.

Do #12

Fill Your Grocery Cart with Farm-Fresh Foods

The other day, I walked into two food stores to see how many foods they had that were *actually* food. Many of the food items you find in your supermarket today are not *real* food. C'mon, you suspected that, didn't you? Real foods grow in the ground, can be picked from a tree, or once walked the earth. Vegetables, fruits, grains, nuts, and meats are real farm-fresh foods. These foods should take up most of the space in your grocery cart. As food activist and writer, Michael Pollan, said in his book, *Food Rules*, everything he learned about food and health can be summed up in these seven words: "Eat food, not too much, mostly plants."

Processed foods, like most breakfast cereals and frozen entrees, chips, Cheese-whiz, Coca Cola, Ding-Dongs, and anything with a string of chemical additives on the label, are not real foods. They are manufactured foods. Manufactured and processed foods are full of chemicals, additives, and preservatives. Chemicals in our food have been linked to many health problems, from heart disease, cancer, and obesity to infertility and mental disorders. These foods are also loaded with fat, sugar, and salt, which also make them perfect little bombs of concentrated calories.

At the beginning of this section, I said: *By choosing healthier foods, you're choosing a healthier life.* Eating "real food" is one of the healthiest choices you can make.

Quick-Starts

☐ **Buy what's in season and locally produced like apples, spinach, kale, cheeses, whole grain breads** and other healthy, fresh foods you find at a farmer's market. They will usually be cheaper and fresher.

☐ **Cut back on foods that contain a long list of ingredients.** Some dietary experts say to eat foods with fewer than five ingredients, particularly when you can't pronounce them.

Your Choice of More How-To's

☐ Ask at your grocery store, "What fruits and vegetables just came in today?" Buy these, they will be the freshest and most nutritious.

☐ If nothing looks fresh in the fruit and produce aisle, head over to the frozen foods section and choose "fresh frozen" vegetables and fruit. Since most supermarket produce is picked before it's ripe, and sits in warehouses before ever making it to your supermarket shelf, they either lose nutrients or never get the chance to develop all their vitamins and minerals. Frozen foods picked and packed at their peak of freshness will be more nutrient-packed.

☐ Shop along the outside aisles of the supermarket where you'll generally find fruits and vegetables, dairy, and meats. Look in the interior aisles for other "real foods" like beans and 100 percent whole grains.

☐ Join a local food co-op if you're lucky enough to have one near you.

☐ Make at least one third of most of your meals vegetables. You might have to work slowly toward this, but your body will thank you. The simplest way to prepare vegetables is to simply cut and steam them for about five minutes. For flavor, add a little salt or salt substitute made from fresh herbs such as A. Vogel Herbamare. Or use low-sodium soy sauce, pepper, mustard, salsa or a dollop of red pepper or artichoke dip. Choose the salsa and dips with the fewest ingredients.

☐ Avoid foods that contain high fructose corn syrup. You'll find this ingredient in many products including sodas, fruit-flavored drinks, bread, and most processed foods. Eating high fructose corn syrup may promote inflammation and obesity.

☐ Favor flavorful whole foods that offer fullness. For the same amount of carbohydrates (15 grams), you can either enjoy 1¼ *cups* of delicious and sweet fresh strawberries or 1½ *tablespoons* of strawberry preserves. I know which I'd choose.

☐ Add more herbs and spices to your cooking. Pepper, cinnamon, oregano, basil, turmeric (found in mustard), parsley, ginger, garlic, and vanilla are all high in healthy, inflammation-fighting anti-oxidants.

Do #13

Become a Label Maven: Check Carbohydrates, Fat, Sodium, and Fiber

If you can read but you're not reading food labels, I'm keeping you after class! For your own sake, get in the habit of reading the Nutrition Facts label found on most packaged foods and beverages. This is vital information that can help you follow your meal plan and stay within your daily number of calories, fats, carbohydrates, and sodium (found in salt).

Sodium makes up 40 percent of salt and has been linked to high blood pressure, strokes, and kidney disease, conditions many people with type 2 diabetes have or are at risk for. When looking at fats, don't just look at Total Fat but also Saturated Fat and Trans Fat. Stay away from Trans Fat. And to see how much a food will raise your blood sugar, check the Total Carbohydrate grams—not the Sugars. Every gram of *both* sugar and starch raises your blood sugar.

Fiber is also on the Nutrition Facts label under Total Carbohydrate. Fiber is the indigestible part of plant foods. It's found in fruits, vegetables, whole grains, nuts, and legumes. When you consume dietary fiber, most of it passes through the intestines and doesn't get digested. Many dietitians recommend subtracting half the fiber grams (if over

5 grams) in a food from the carbohydrate count when counting your carbs. For example, if a serving of whole wheat pasta has 37 carbohydrates and 6 grams of fiber, subtract 3 (half of 6) from 37 and consider 34 carbohydrates as your carb intake. If a food contains fewer than 5 grams of fiber per serving, don't subtract any carbs from the carb count.

Remember, food grams are given in "Amount Per Serving." If you intend to eat twice the serving size, like having two slices of bread instead of one, you have to double the carbohydrate grams on the package label. Even if you don't intend to, but end up doing it anyway, you don't get to slide on this one.

Quick-Starts

☐ **Read the list of ingredients on food packages before you drop them in your shopping cart.** Know that the first ingredient listed is what the product contains the most of. Then decide if it still goes in your cart.

☐ **When reading labels don't be fooled.** "Sugar" can show up under several names such as sucrose, fructose, glucose, dextrose, lactose, maltose, raw sugar, corn syrup, high fructose corn syrup, honey, maple syrup, molasses, and evaporated cane juice. These are all forms of sugar.

Your Choice of More How-To's

☐ Ask your health care provider, diabetes educator, or a dietitian how many carbohydrates you should eat at each meal and the amount of calories, fats, and sodium you should have in a day.

☐ Be aware that a health claim on a food's label doesn't necessarily mean it's healthy. Diet cola is "100% fat-free" but it doesn't contain any health benefits. "Low-fat" often means there's more sugar in a product. The only way to know what you're getting for sure is to read the Nutrition Facts label.

☐ Read the label on protein bars like Zone, Clif Bar, Kashi, Kind, and Nature Valley. Many are high in carbohydrates and some have as many calories as a candy bar.

☐ To help you keep track of the carbohydrates, fats, and calories in foods you eat regularly, cut out their nutrition labels and keep them in a scrapbook or photo album.

☐ Carbohydrates on a package's label are allowed to be up to 20 percent off, so if you want to really see what a food does to your blood sugar, check on your meter before and two hours after you eat it.

Counting carbohydrates and carbohydrate exchanges:

• Two systems for knowing how much medication to take for what you eat are counting carbohydrates and using the exchange system. If you take insulin, you should have an insulin-to-carbohydrate ratio. In other words, one unit of insulin for you will cover approximately a certain number of carbs. The general rule of thumb is one unit of insulin covers 15 grams of carbs, but it may be different for you. If you're using the carbohydrate exchange system, 15 grams of carbohydrates in a food is considered one carbohydrate exchange.

• Since most foods don't contain carbs in multiples of fifteen, carbohydrate exchanges are given based on ranges. If a food contains fewer than 5 grams of carbs, the exchange value is zero. Foods containing 6 to 10 grams of carbohydrates are considered one-half a carbohydrate exchange. Foods containing 11 to 20 grams of carbohydrates are considered one carbohydrate exchange.

• These foods contain 11 to 20 grams of carbs and are considered one carbohydrate exchange:

   ○ 1 slice of bread

   ○ 1 flour or corn tortilla (6 inch)

   ○ ¼ of a bagel

   ○ 1 pancake

   ○ ¾ cup of most cold breakfast cereals

○ ⅓ cup of cooked rice or pasta

○ ¼ of a large baked potato

○ 3 graham crackers

○ 6 saltines

○ 3 cups of popcorn

○ ¾ cup plain yogurt

○ 1 small fruit

○ 2 small cookies

○ 1 envelope of hot chocolate

○ 5 chocolate kisses

• You can find more information on carbohydrate counting on the American Diabetes Association website at diabetes.org/food-and-fitness/food/planning-meals/carb-counting.

Do #14

Graze—It's Good for You!

There's much to be said for eating five or six small meals throughout the day instead of three big meals. The benefits stack up like this:

1. It helps keep you from getting the munchies in between meals because you're always somewhat full.
2. It can keep your blood sugar more level throughout the day.
3. It boosts your metabolism to burn more calories.
4. It may keep your cells from storing fat.
5. You'll have more energy because your body is getting a constant supply of fuel.
6. Your digestive system won't be overworked trying to process lots of food all at once.
7. You won't feel deprived because you know you'll be putting something into your mouth again soon. Now, now...

At the University of Cambridge, researchers discovered that eating less food more often is also good for your heart. People who ate six small meals a day, rather than two large meals, lowered their cholesterol levels by 5 percent.

Just be alert not to let grazing become an excuse to eat whatever you want whenever you want. Portion control is essential when you graze.

Quick-Starts

☐ **Keep your last and next graze about two and a half to three hours apart** unless you're sleeping.

☐ **Eat about the same amount of carbohydrates for most meals and snacks** to keep your blood sugar more level.

Your Choice of More How-To's

☐ Fruit, raw vegetables, string cheese, nuts, and a small container of yogurt or cottage cheese make portable, healthy snacks. I also nibble on a few cherry or grape tomatoes. Tomatoes are actually a fruit and these little gobbles are sweet and delicious.

☐ When I'm at home, I often snack in between meals on a hard boiled egg or a few slices of thinly sliced turkey breast you get at the deli counter of a supermarket. Protein is an excellent filler-upper.

☐ Drink plenty of water throughout the day.

☐ Work with your health care provider, or a dietitian or diabetes educator, to create a meal and snack plan that meets your needs.

Here's a sample menu to give you an idea of what six meals/snacks a day looks like:

• 7:30 AM — One serving of oatmeal (don't forget mine! See "Do #11. Turn Ho-Hum Oatmeal into your 'Can't-Wait-For' Breakfast.") with a sprinkle of sunflower or pumpkin seeds and bite-sized pieces from half an apple, peach, plum, or pear; coffee or tea

- 10 AM – 6 ounces of plain yogurt topped with a tablespoon of chopped walnuts
- 12:30 PM – Spinach salad with veggies, canned salmon packed in water, a light olive oil and vinegar dressing, three whole-wheat crackers (I prefer Finn Crisp and Wasa for their low carbohydrate count yet full flavor) and half a banana
- 3 PM – 1 cup raw veggies with ¼ cup hummus
- 6 PM – 3 ounces grilled chicken breast (the size of your palm), 2 cups steamed broccoli drizzled with a little olive oil, ½ cup cooked brown rice, and a small bowl of berries for dessert
- 8 PM – 3 cups of light microwave or air-popped popcorn or half an apple with a tablespoon of peanut butter

Do #15

When Drinking, Keep Your Blood Sugar from Sinking

I love wine and I often have a glass, occasionally two, at night with dinner. For years I couldn't figure out why it lowered my blood sugar—so here's the scoop. While I'm sure there's a better way to say this medically, the liver gets busy processing the alcohol from the wine, so it doesn't release glucose (sugar) into the blood stream as it normally would. Boom, your blood sugar drops. This is true if you're drinking any pure alcohol like vodka, gin, scotch, bourbon, rye, and wine. If you drink, it's really important to watch that your blood sugar doesn't go too low. It can, and most people I know who use insulin have a scary story to tell about it.

On the other hand, most cocktails, particularly those that you're embarrassed to call by name (multiple screaming orgasm, fuzzy navel, salty chihuahua, mudslide, side car, zombie, or even your cosmopolitan), will raise your blood sugar because they contain some form of sugar. Cocktails tend to contain sugary mixers like soda, fruit juice, tonic, or sweetened lemon/lime mix. You'll find these in screwdrivers, greyhounds, salty dogs, sea breezes, mojitos, rum and cokes, daiquiris, margaritas, pina coladas, and more. As for liqueurs, these will send your blood sugar into the stratosphere. While I like Sambuca and Frangelico as much as the next person, my blood sugar definitely doesn't.

Also be aware that alcohol is high in calories (1 gram of alcohol contains 7 calories) and has few nutrients. A typical 5 ounce glass of wine contains approximately 100 calories. A typical 12 ounce light beer contains the same 100 calories. A regular 12 ounce beer contains about 150 calories. Drinking is a very easy way to put on weight. We don't tend to think about the calories in liquids, and once you start drinking, you won't be as clear-headed to watch what you're consuming.

That lack of clear-headedness can also make you unaware that your blood sugar is dropping, or how much it's already dropped. It can be easy to miss the signs and symptoms of low blood sugar (see "Do #35. Be Prepared for Hypoglycemia"). It may also appear that you are drunk even when you're not. Slurring your words, seeming "out of it" and becoming irritable, anxious, or aggressive can all be signs of low blood sugar. Make sure at least one of your drinking companions knows that you have diabetes, and if you look like you're drunk it may be that your blood sugar is too low and you need some carbohydrate (half a glass of juice, regular soda, or a glucose drink or tablets). Lastly, if you have a seizure or pass out, someone should call 911 right away.

Drinking can be fun. Drinking can also be dangerous, especially if you take insulin or another glucose-lowering medication. Drink in moderation and ask your doctor if your medication puts you at risk for low blood sugar while drinking. To be safe, watch your consumption and make sure you carry your meter and some form of sugar with you.

Quick-Starts

☐ **If you're not going to order food and there are crackers, pretzels, or chips on the bar, eat some if you're drinking a drink that will drop your blood sugar.** Don't overdo it, however, or you can raise your blood sugar too much, and you'll be adding calories that can pack on the pounds. *Tip:* Nuts won't raise your blood sugar very much.

☐ **If you're going out for a drink, carry glucose tablets with you.**
If your blood sugar goes below 70 mg/dl (3.8 mmol/l), you will want
to raise it quickly.

Your Choice of More How-To's

☐ Always inform someone you're drinking with that you have diabetes.
Tell them the signs of low blood sugar and that if you exhibit those signs
to make sure you drink half a glass of juice or regular soda to bring up
your blood sugar. Tell them also to call 911 if you start behaving oddly
or pass out, and to say on the phone that you have diabetes.

☐ Eat something that will raise your blood sugar before you go for a
drink so it won't drop too low while you're drinking.

☐ If there's no food at the bar, see if they will serve you some bread so
your blood sugar doesn't drop too low.

☐ If you're drinking and not eating, remember to take less medication. I don't need any insulin if I'm drinking wine and eating very few
carbohydrates.

☐ If your drink has carbohydrates in it, like juice or a sweet mixer, or
you're drinking beer, count it in your total carbohydrate intake. For
example, two beers contain about 13 grams of carbs each, so you would
count this as two carb choices (a carbohydrate choice has approximately
15 grams of carbohydrate) or 26 grams of carbs.

☐ Know if your medication doesn't mix well with alcohol. For example,
glucophage (Metformin) is not recommended if you typically consume
more than two drinks a day. Discuss this with your doctor if it affects you.

How to handle sleeping after drinking:

• Always check your blood sugar before going to sleep. If you are low, eat some carbohydrates and a little protein to bring up your blood sugar. I also have a few bites of Extend Bar. It helps keep blood sugar level for seven to nine hours.

• Check your blood sugar before you drink and before you go to sleep to see how much alcohol drops it in those few hours. One glass of wine doesn't lower my blood sugar but two definitely does.

• Check your blood sugar before you go to sleep and set your alarm and do a 3 AM check to see where your blood sugar is. This is around the time your blood sugar may be plummeting. Raise your blood sugar with some glucose tablets or half a glass of juice or some other fast-acting sugar if it's below or just above 70 mg/dl (3.8 mmol/l) so it won't drop lower before you wake up.

Do #16

Eat from 9-Inch Dinner Plates

Dine on smaller plates and you may soon delight in a smaller waist. You can cut up to 35 percent of your daily calories by swapping your 12-inch dinner plates for 9-inch ones, according to the authors of the book, *The 9-Inch Diet*. You may not know it, but today's average plate size has expanded, inviting us to load up on one-third more food than people did twenty years ago.

Lest you think you'll feel deprived, Brian Wansink, author of *Mindless Eating*, says studies show that we tend to eat 92 percent of what we're served, regardless of how much we're served. And since we all like statistics, Cornell University researchers ran a study and discovered that putting your food on a smaller plate can help you lose eighteen pounds in a year! Yes, I like that statistic.

Quick-Starts

☐ **Measure your lunch and dinner plates.** If you eat off a plate larger than ten inches, pick up enough plates for you and your family that are nine or ten inches.

☐ **Use taller, thinner drinking glasses.** Cornell University research shows that drinking liquids out of taller, thinner glasses makes us think we are drinking more than we actually are.

Your Choice of More How-To's

☐ Use plates that are not too small. Wansink's research shows that if you switch to plates that are *too* small, like salad plates, you'll know you're skimping and may be tempted to pile up helpings or go back for more.

☐ Use round rather than square plates. A 10-inch square plate has about 21 square inches more surface area than a 10-inch round plate!

☐ When you get a dish in a restaurant that comes on a big platter or in a big bowl, ask your server for a smaller plate. Portion out half and take the other half home.

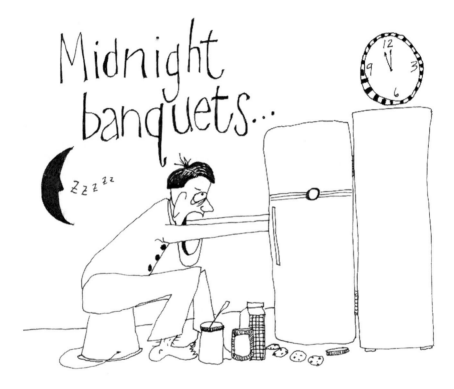

Do #17

Savor "Must Have" Treats When You Must

Who thought never having a cookie or a piece of cheesecake again was actually going to happen just because you got diabetes?! The good news is there's no reason why it should. The American Diabetes Association says sweets are fine if they're eaten in moderation. That means you can indulge now and then in a small portion of your favorites. Unless, of course, there's a medical reason why you shouldn't. I'm addicted to dark chocolate and halvah (a sweet made of ground sesame seeds, tahini, and sugar or honey). A few times a week I have one or two small squares of dark chocolate and a sliver (very small slice) of halvah as my nighttime treat.

If you see a diabetes educator or work with a dietitian, plan your indulgences into a weekly meal plan. Knowing they're coming in a day or two may make it easier to resist temptation on any one day. Well, except perhaps when your favorite team loses the Super Bowl!

What you need to know is that sweets are concentrated calories and offer little to no nutritional value. As you get more serious about your health and the nutrition of your foods, you may want to keep cutting back on processed sweets until they are pretty much out of your diet.

That said, having *occasional* treats may keep you from feeling deprived and help you stick to your meal plan. Dr. Dean Ornish, founder of the Preventive Medicine Research Institute, says when your diet is mostly healthy foods you can allow yourself to indulge in the "yummy stuff" now and then. Of course, he probably wasn't including midnight banquets.

Quick-Starts

☐ **If it's after 8 PM, have a smaller size serving of your treat,** such as one small scoop of ice cream, one or two small squares of chocolate, or one cookie.

☐ **If you go overboard on a treat,** eat slightly less food the next day or skip a sweet that may be planned for that day.

Your Choice of More How-To's

☐ Small portions of treats now and then are the key to enjoying sweets and reducing the sugars, fats, and calories you eat.

☐ To stop a binge in its tracks, change your flavor palette. If I've just eaten two squares of my favorite dark chocolate and think I'm about to devour the whole bar, I put it back in the pantry and eat an olive. The saltiness stops the sweet craving!

☐ If you overindulge, don't beat yourself up. Even if you've been off the rails for days. Just get back on your meal plan now.

☐ Keep your favorites in the freezer. You can usually find part of a blueberry oatmeal scone and a few chocolate biscotti in mine. They last longer this way, and since I forget they're there half the time, I only munch on them occasionally. *Tip:* If you put a scone, muffin or big cookie in the freezer, break it into pieces first. That way you can just defrost and eat one piece rather than the whole thing.

Do #18

Keep a Food Diary and Double Your Weight Loss

Get this: write down everything you eat for one month and you're likely to lose weight. No, it's not the calories you're burning writing. Kaiser Permanente's Center for Health Research conducted one of the largest and longest weight-loss trials ever, including 1,680 overweight men and women ages twenty-five and up for a period of twenty weeks. They discovered that people who kept daily food records lost twice as much weight as those who didn't.

It turns out just the act of scribbling down what you eat, even on a sticky note, makes you more aware of what you eat. How many of us count the number of potato chips or pretzels we eat when we've got the bag on our lap? Or the handfuls of salty peanuts we grab each time we pass the tin? Or how many cups of pasta are actually in that beautiful Italian ceramic bowl at your favorite Italian restaurant? Studies show when you notice what's going into your mouth, you're likely to take more responsibility for what you put in there.

Quick-Starts

☐ **For just three days, record everything you eat and drink and how much.** Do it as you eat and drink, not at the end of the day when you're tired or may forget. Calculate the amount of what you eat and drink by size like a 2" x 1" piece of cheese, or by amount like ½ cup of peas, or by weight like 8 ounces of chocolate milk. Everything counts, including sauces and gravies, salad dressing, soda, butter, mayonnaise, and even a piece of sucking candy or a few pretzels. If you can do it longer, go for a week.

☐ **Review your food log at the end of the day and see if you notice anything. Compare your three day results and see what you notice.** For instance, do you always seem to snack at 10 AM? If so, keep a piece of fruit nearby for when that hunger strikes. It may just stop you from raiding the pantry for cupcakes.

Your Choice of More How-To's

☐ If you want to go a step further with your food log, counting calories can be a tool to help you see just how many you're eating. The general recommendation is for women to eat 1,600–2,200 calories a day and for men, 2,400–3,000 calories a day, depending upon age and activity. Estimate the calories in everything you eat and drink and write them down. You'll discover whether you're really staying within your caloric allowance or not. Just seeing this calorie count is likely to help you eat a little less during the day if you're over your calorie limit. Having said that, bear in mind whether you spend 1,000 calories on soda, or apples and broccoli, makes a difference in how much disease-fighting nutrition you're getting, and whether your body stores those calories as ready-to-use-fuel or as fat.

☐ Think about why you eat what you do, and when. You may discover much of your eating is for emotional comfort, boredom, frustration, or restlessness, not hunger. If so, see if you can replace some of that eating with an activity you enjoy. When I'm creeping toward the fridge, it often works for me to change what I'm doing, like getting out and taking a short walk.

Ways to keep a log:

• If you prefer to write your log, choose a small, thin notebook. It will be easier to carry with you at all times.

• You can choose from a number of websites to help keep your food journal on your computer. Here are a few: myfooddiary.com, fitday.com, and livestrong.com/thedailyplate.

• Keep a food diary on your smartphone. A few apps for mobile devices include: dLife Diabetes Companion, Weight Watchers Mobile, MyNetDiary, Fat Secret, and iFoodDiary.

Do #19

Stay on Track Despite Holiday Temptations

Ah, it's the holidays. So anticipated and yet so dreaded. But I've got a plan to help you avoid that typical five to ten pound holiday weight gain. This plan has two parts. Part one: indulge in whatever you want to eat. Part two: expect to lose no weight from Thanksgiving to New Years. In fact, you may even gain a pound or two. But not the usual ten. By nibbling on the things you want to eat—two tiny puff pastries, not eighteen—you may keep yourself from feeling deprived and like you need to veer completely off your meal plan.

So ration holiday foods, but don't eliminate them. Trust me, come January you'll be mighty pleased to be enjoying the healthy rewards of sticking (mostly) to your meal plan.

Quick-Starts

☐ **Go to a party with something in your stomach.** Eat a healthy snack before you go, like a piece of fruit, some raw veggies and hummus, a hard boiled egg, a serving of string cheese, a salad with olive oil and vinegar, or a small handful of unsalted nuts.

☐ **Eat three meals a day or smaller more frequent meals.** If you skip meals, you can end up eating more calories than you would by eating regular meals. Most people who skip meals take in extra calories snacking at night when hunger catches up with them.

Your Choice of More How-To's

☐ Be a little more physically active during the holidays to burn extra calories.

☐ Drink water before and after a glass of alcohol to cut your alcohol intake.

☐ Slow down your eating and drinking by savoring textures and tastes.

☐ Put fifteen feet between you and the food table when you're at a party.

☐ When the finger food is passed around, ignore the servers half of the time. Trust me, they won't take it personally.

☐ When you entertain, give any extra food away to your guests.

☐ When you're not entertaining, keep those pretty bowls of sweets off the coffee table.

Do #20

Limit Fast Food—Or You'll Be "Fat Fast!"

Most foods you find at a fast food joint or local chain restaurant are fat-bombs. Think Double Quarter Pounder with cheese, super-sized French fries and sodas, double-dipped chicken teriyaki, Buffalo wings, and glazed onion rings. The same goes for many foods at the corner deli like giant-sized muffins, salads dripping in ranch dressing, and deli spreads loaded with mayo. Eating too many of these foods quickly adds up to thousands more calories than is healthy. Plus, because these fried and processed foods are packed with fat, sugar, and salt, they're an invitation not just to weight gain, but also high blood pressure and high cholesterol. And these are conditions many people with type 2 diabetes already have or are at risk for.

Dr. Michael Roizen, Dr. Mehmet Oz's writing partner and Chief Wellness Officer at the famous Cleveland Clinic says, "You can't make a deal with food!" What we eat either turns on our genes for disease or not. The good news is we get to control what we eat.

If you grab your meals and snacks on the run, slow down long enough to read the whole menu and make healthier choices more often. Now you actually have that option since many fast food and chain restaurants offer healthier items.

Quick-Starts

☐ **Choose smaller sizes at fast food restaurants.** Stick to the regular, small, or kiddie-size French fries, hamburgers, soda, and/or bag of chips. Super-sizing doubles and triples a food's calories, fat, sugar, and salt.

☐ **If you work outside your home, bring your lunch to work at least a few times a week** rather than go out and buy it.

Your Choice of More How-To's

☐ Set a limit on how often you eat fast food, like once a week or twice a month if you eat it more often now.

☐ Go easy on the sauces. Don't pour them on but use a spoon to dribble just enough on for flavor. Most contain a good deal of sugar, fat, salt, and calories.

☐ Resist overeating side dishes or grabbing a pack of chips, cookies, or a giant soda because you feel you deserve them after choosing a healthy entrée.

☐ When you enter a fast food or chain restaurant, look to see if calories are posted or listed on the menu. Think about which choices will satisfy both your taste and your waist.

☐ If you can't drive by the donut shop without stopping, change your route.

A round up of healthier choices on fast food menus:

• At Subway, get a 6" sandwich or salad. The Footlong sandwich starts at 540 calories and can have more salt than the daily recommended allowance of 1500 milligrams.

• Taco Bell offers a Fresco Style Grilled Steak Soft Taco for 170 calories and 5 grams of fat. Or try the Chicken Gordita Nacho Cheese for 270 calories and 10 grams of fat.

• At McDonalds, choose an Egg McMuffin over a sausage, egg and cheese McGriddle. You'll save 250 calories, 20 grams of fat and 400 mg of sodium (salt).

• At IHOP, choose the tomato, spinach, and mushroom omelet for 350 calories instead of the pancakes and garden omelet entrée for 1,240 calories.

• At Dunkin Donuts, don't get suckered into a fat-free item. These almost always are higher in sugar than the item they're replacing. Choose an egg sandwich for under 300 calories. If your craving for a donut is causing you to break into a sweat, choose a plain sugar coated donut. At 260 calories, it has almost half the calories of the apple crumb donut.

• At Ruby Tuesday, you can enjoy a full steak dinner (7oz. sirloin, green beans, and sautéed mushrooms) for less than half the calories of a turkey burger and fries.

• At Starbucks, a grande brewed coffee contains about 5 calories and a few more if you add cream and sugar. A 16-ounce nonfat latte has 160 calories. But look at these other drinks: Those sweet summery frozen drinks, like Java Chip Frappuccino, weigh in with 650 calories and 25 grams of fat—50 calories more than a Big Mac! The grande caffe vanilla Frappucino contains 64 grams of sugar! And that lovely warming hot chocolate in the dark of winter, with 2 percent milk and whipped cream, contains 370 calories, 16 grams of fat, and 40 grams of sugar! The American Diabetes Association recommends women get no more than 100 calories (25 grams) in added sugar in a day and men no more than 150 (37 grams). Choose wisely.

• Au Bon Pain has eliminated trans fat from all its cookies, bagels, and muffins, and California Pizza Kitchen is in the process of doing the same. Ruby Tuesday is deep-frying its foods in heart-healthy canola oil. Yet Popeyes and Friendly's still serve foods with unhealthy trans fats.

• "Stop & Go Fast Food Nutrition Guide" lists the calories, fat, cholesterol, sodium, and carbs from more than sixty fast food and chain restaurants like Applebee's, Cici's Pizza, Denny's, Hardee's, KFC, Long John Silver's, O'Charley's, Panda Express, and Popeyes. You can find it at maplemountainpress.com/ffg_form.php.

Shared Learning

Since we learn from each other, here are some personal "How-To's" from people living with diabetes:

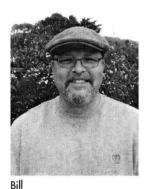

I am of Latin heritage, and my mom is from Cuba. We eat rice and beans with everything! As of late, if I choose to eat beans, I make that my protein and skip the meat. This cuts down on my fat intake, too.

— **Bill Rodriguez**
49 years old, living with diabetes 35 years.

Bill

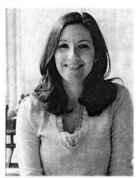

I manage to eat healthy by making substitutions. I love hummus and pita. When I don't want to eat added carbs, I use endive leaves instead of pita chips. They also work fantastically for salsa and guacamole plus they look really pretty!

— **Elizabeth Edelman**
30 years old, living with diabetes 7 years.

Elizabeth

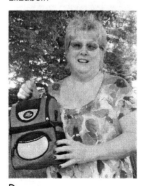

My little red cooler goes everywhere I go so I can always eat something healthy. At different times, my cooler is filled with fresh fruit, yogurt, trail mix, almonds, celery with hummus on it, butter rum candies, mixed fruit in its own juices, fresh cut pineapple, veggies with lite ranch dressing, 100 calorie cookies, egg salad, mixed greens, and sunflower seeds. I make different choices so I don't get tired of eating the same things and I never leave home without my little red cooler!

— **Doreen Bugai**
57 years old, living with diabetes 36 years.

Doreen

Your Quick-Start "Do" Sheet

Use this worksheet to help you accomplish any Food "Do" in a way that works best for you.

The "Do" I will do is:

_____

_____

_____

Why it's important to me to do this:

_____

_____

_____

My "How-To" is/are:

_____

_____

_____

When I will begin:

_____

_____

_____

How often I will do this:

_____

_____

_____

Where I will do this:

_____

_____

_____

Who can support me:

_____

_____

_____

What can stop me:

_____

_____

_____

What I will do about that:

_____

_____

_____

What was successful and how I can keep doing it:

_____

_____

_____

Medical Do's

Medical stuff is in this section.
Don't worry, we'll get through it together.

I hope clear, vinyl handbags NEVER come back in style.

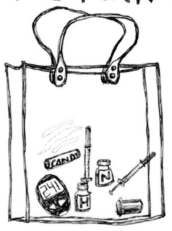

Do #21

Learn Your Diabetes A-B-C's

Managing diabetes well requires you to know a great deal about diabetes, and yourself, and put that knowledge to good use. I truly believe knowledge is powerful medicine. Years ago, after reading that newer insulins existed that might help me better control my blood sugar, I went to a certified diabetes educator. She switched me from my older insulins to a newer rapid- and long-acting insulin that gives me much better control.

Some essentials to know for managing your diabetes are called "Diabetes A-B-C's." "A" stands for your Hemoglobin A1C. This is usually just called A1C. An A1C is a measurement that shows your blood sugar average over the past two to three months. For an A1C test, you typically have your blood drawn either at your doctor's office or a lab. Your A1C gives you and your doctor an idea of how well managed your blood sugar is and if your treatment plan is working for you.

"B" stands for blood pressure. Many people with type 2 diabetes have high blood pressure. High blood pressure is also called the "silent killer" because you may not feel anything. "C" stands for cholesterol. If you have high cholesterol, as do many people with type 2 diabetes, you may be more likely to get a heart attack or stroke. Nearly 65 percent of people with type 2 diabetes die from heart attack or stroke.

Here are some tools to help you beat those odds. Below are the standard guidelines and target ranges recommended for most people with diabetes. That said, you're not most people with diabetes, you're you. So ask your doctor if these should be your target ranges, too. I can't stress this enough. In fact, guidelines for health care professionals this year encourage more individualized treatment goals. So take a look at the general recommendations below—and then find out what *your* numbers should be.

Hemoglobin A1C: Less than 6.5–7%. People with hypoglycemic unawareness (don't feel the symptoms of low blood sugar), or some other conditions, may be advised to keep their A1C slightly higher than the recommendation.

Quick-Starts A1C

☐ **If you don't know your A1C, call your doctor and schedule an A1C test.** Then be sure you discuss the result with him and what to do about it.

☐ **If you do know your A1C and it's above 7%** discuss with your doctor if this is appropriate for you, and if not, how to bring it down. No matter how high it is, bringing it down just one percent can reduce your risk of getting diabetes complications (see "Do #22. Know How to Delay or Prevent Diabetes Complications.") If you need to bring it down, work on bringing it down one percent, then one more percent, then one more percent. You get the idea.

Blood pressure: Less than 130/80 mmHg (17.3/10.6 kPa)

Quick-Starts Blood Pressure

☐ **Ask your doctor to take your blood pressure at every visit.** If it's too high, discuss ways to bring it down.

☐ **Buy an over-the-counter blood pressure cuff at a pharmacy or home medical supply store** and check your blood pressure at home. I have the Omron Intelli-sense® at home. If you have more than three high readings in a row taken on separate days, tell your health care provider.

What to do before a blood pressure reading:

- Wear short sleeves so your arm is exposed.

- Don't drink coffee or smoke at least thirty minutes beforehand.

- Use the bathroom before having your blood pressure taken. Having to go can affect your reading.

- Keep your legs uncrossed and your feet flat on the floor.

Total Cholesterol: Generally advised to be less than 180–200 mg/dl (below 5.2 mmol/l). But much more important is your HDL and LDL cholesterol, which make up your total cholesterol.

- HDL ("Healthy" cholesterol): In men, higher than 40 mg/dl (1 mmol/l). In women, higher than 50 mg/dl (1.3 mmol/l).

- LDL ("Lousy" cholesterol): Lower than 100 mg/dl (2.6 mmol/l) if you have no pre-existing heart disease and less than 70 mg/dl (1.8 mmol/l) if you do have heart disease or are at risk for heart disease.

- Triglycerides: Less than 150 mg/dl (1.7 mmol/l).

Quick-Starts Cholesterol

☐ **Have your cholesterol measured (simple blood test at a lab) at least once a year.** If your LDL is too high, or your HDL too low, sometimes a diet of mostly vegetables, fruit, whole grains, lean meats, nuts, and seeds may improve these numbers. That said, many experts believe dietary cholesterol (foods you eat that contain cholesterol) have little impact on your cholesterol.

☐ **Add fish oil to your diet by taking a fish oil supplement.** You can take fish oil in pills which you'll find in your local health food store. Fish oil is an anti-inflammatory that has been shown to lower LDL cholesterol and triglycerides and may have a positive effect on HDL cholesterol. As healthy as this sounds, discuss it first with your health care provider.

Your Choice of More How-To's

☐ If you have type 1 diabetes, get an A1C test every three months. If you have type 2 diabetes and your A1C is not where your doctor wants it to be (yuk!), you should also get an A1C test every three months. If your A1C is routinely below 7%, get an A1C test every six months.

☐ Many people find they gain more control when they log their blood sugar, medication, food, and exercise. If you'd like to try, the free Glucose Buddy diabetes tracking app is one of the most widely used.

☐ A type of medicine called statins help lower LDL cholesterol when diet cannot. Statins are also protective for people who have already had a heart attack. But statins may also come with side effects. Talk with your health care provider and see if statins are a good option for you.

☐ If you take a statin and do experience side effects, CoQ10, a health supplement you can find in health food stores, may reduce some side effects of statins. Ask your health care provider about taking this.

☐ While not routine, there's a new cholesterol test called NMR. This test checks the number and size of your cholesterol particles. Currently there's a lot of debate whether it's number of particles, or size, that plays the bigger role in cardiovascular risk.

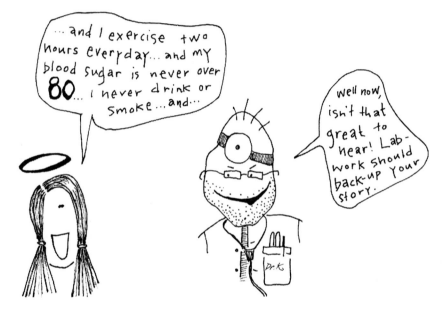

Do #22

Know How to Delay or Prevent Diabetes Complications

Diabetes complications are caused by high blood sugars that over time—usually years—slowly damage the large and small blood vessels in your body. This damage affects the circulatory, nerve, and digestive systems, and most parts of your body including your brain, heart, kidney, eyes, hands, feet, and legs. High blood pressure and high cholesterol also damage blood vessels, so you want to also keep your blood pressure and cholesterol in check (see "Do #21. Learn Your Diabetes A-B-C's.")

The most common diabetes complications include:

- cardiovascular (heart) disease

- neuropathy (nerve damage) in feet, legs, and hands

- foot ulcer and foot amputation from a foot infection

- retinopathy (eye disease), including blindness

- periodontal (gum) disease

- nephropathy (kidney) disease

Less common complications include gastroparesis (slow stomach emptying), trigger fingers, frozen shoulders, sexual dysfunction including erectile dysfunction, hearing loss, birth defects, Alzheimer's, and dementia. Because type 1 diabetes is an autoimmune condition, people with type 1 may be genetically predisposed to other autoimmune conditions like Hashimoto's disease (under-active thyroid), Grave's disease (over-active thyroid), and celiac disease (can't tolerate gluten found in wheat, rye, and barley).

The single best way to reduce your risk of diabetes complications is to keep your blood sugars within your target range as much as is humanly possible. The general recommendation from the American Diabetes Association (ADA): blood sugar between 70 and 130 mg/dl (3.8–7.2 mmol/l) when you first wake up in the morning and before meals, and less than 180 mg/dl (10 mmol/l) two hours after a meal. The American Association of Clinical Endocrinologists (AACE) recommends somewhat lower targets: less than 110 mg/dl (6.1 mmol/l) before meals and less than 140 mg/dl (7.7 mmol/l) two hours after a meal. Discuss what is best for you with your health care provider.

You may get the idea that diabetes complications are not something you want to have happen to you—and you'd be right. But remember what I first said—when you hear "heart attack," "amputation," "kidney disease," and "blindness" mentioned in the same sentence as "diabetes," it isn't just having diabetes that causes these, but having "poorly controlled" diabetes for several years.

You have a certain amount of power over your health. Keep your blood sugar in your target range most of the time, and control your blood pressure and cholesterol, and you will be less likely to suffer complications. Also know that many people live a full and productive life with few complications.

Quick-Starts

☐ **Always take your medicines when and as directed.** If you don't know how much to take or when, call your doctor. Skipping your medicine much of the time will make you more vulnerable to getting complications.

☐ **Ask your health care provider what target range she recommends for your blood sugar, blood pressure, and cholesterol.** Be sure you understand how to get to, and stay in, these ranges.

Your Choice of More How-To's

☐ Eat healthy, maintain a normal weight, be physically active, and don't smoke. These actions will help keep your blood sugar, blood pressure, and cholesterol within your target range.

☐ Have your lab tests done a week or two before your doctor appointment. This way you can discuss your results. Always ask what actions you can take to improve any test result that needs improving.

☐ Bring your doctor a record of your blood sugars taken over a few weeks. Good times to check your blood sugar are when you wake up, before meals, and two hours after you begin a meal. With this record, your doctor can see if your treatment plan needs any tweaking.

☐ Review your treatment plan with your doctor or health care provider at least once a year.

☐ See your health care providers two to four times a year because, at the start of many complications, you won't feel any symptoms. If your blood sugar and/or diabetes is not well managed, or if you use insulin, you should see your doctor every three months.

☐ Some supplements may be helpful if you have complications. Alpha lipoic acid, an anti-oxidant found in health food stores, is often helpful for the tingling or burning sensation of neuropathy usually felt in the feet or legs. I've used it for a tingling in my calf that comes and goes, and found it helpful. Diabetes educators advise 600 mg a day. B vitamins may also be helpful for neuropathy. Always discuss taking supplements with your doctor.

Get these lab tests done regularly:

• An A1C test should be done every three months if your blood sugar is not well controlled and at least every six months if it is.

• Once a year have:

  ○ a blood test to determine your LDL (lousy) and HDL (healthy) cholesterol and triglycerides

  ○ a urine test to check for microalbumin, elevated levels are an early marker for kidney disease

  ○ a serum creatinine and BUN test to check how well your kidneys are working

  ○ a dilated eye exam from an optometrist or ophthalmologist

• Each time you see your doctor, ask him to check your blood pressure and look at your feet.

• Once a year have a full foot exam from a podiatrist (foot specialist), including an ankle brachial ratio, a test that checks for blocked arteries.

• If you have type 1 diabetes, get your thyroid function tested and have a test for celiac disease every year or every other year.

Do #23

Manage Your Blood Sugar Like an Ace Pilot

Did you know that most of the time when an airplane is flying it is actually flying off course? By checking the plane's instruments, the pilot continually directs the plane back on course. In the same way, it's only when we check our blood sugar instruments—our blood glucose meter, continuous glucose monitor if you use one, and A1C test (blood test that measures your blood sugar average over the past two to three months)—and see what our blood sugar is, that we can see whether or not we're on course. In other words, whether our blood sugar is generally within our recommended target range.

The American Diabetes Association (ADA) recommends these target ranges for our blood sugar: between 70 and 130 mg/dl (3.8–7.2 mmol/l) when we first wake up in the morning and before meals, and less than 180 mg/dl (10 mmol/l) two hours after a meal. The American Association of Clinical Endocrinologists (AACE) recommends lower targets. They advise our blood sugar be less than 110 mg/dl (6.1 mmol/l) before meals and less than 140 mg/dl (7.7 mmol/l) two hours after a meal. Personally, I try to keep my blood sugar on the lower scale; I find the less high it goes, the less difficult it is to bring it back down.

If you find your blood sugar is often below and/or above your target range, it's time to make a course correction. Work with your health care provider to make refinements to your treatment plan. Here's one more thing: if you're really working at managing your blood sugar, it's also important to manage your expectations of yourself, and your results. At times they just won't be what you hope for. Even with instruments to help guide us, at times managing diabetes is a bit like flying blind: we can't control our blood sugar with the perfection of a fully functioning pancreas. Do your best, that's all you can ask of yourself.

Quick-Starts

☐ **Wash your hands before you check your blood sugar (and not just because it's sanitary).** If you've just handled food that's sweet, like fruit or barbecue chicken, you can get a higher reading on your meter. Also, thoroughly dry your hands before testing. A wet finger invites a drop of blood to spread, which will make it nearly impossible to get it on your test strip. Then you'll have to do the whole darn poking-your-finger thing again.

☐ **Use the Roche ACCU-CHEK® Testing in Pairs tool.** Seven days in a row check your blood sugar before and two hours after you begin a meal, or before and after you exercise. For instance, check your blood sugar before and after breakfast for a week, then before and after lunch for a week, then before and after dinner for a week. And before and after any regular exercise routine you follow. This type of testing will help you and your doctor see patterns and where you might tweak your treatment plan. To get a paper tool to help you chart your patterns go to accu-chek.com/us/data-management/testing-in-pairs.html.

Your Choice of More How-To's

☐ I can't stress this enough: if you're having difficulty keeping your blood sugar in your target range, talk to your health care provider. If you have type 2 diabetes and you're following your treatment plan, chances are you need a change in medication. Over time, your body may produce less insulin or use it less effectively. If you're already taking several pills, they may just not be powerful enough anymore to keep your blood sugar where it should be. At this point, you'll probably benefit from using insulin or another injectable medicine. Your goal is to keep your blood sugar in your target range as much as possible. That means eating right, being active and taking the right medicine. If you have type 1 diabetes and you're having trouble keeping your blood sugar in target range, your meal plan, activity, and the amount of insulin you take may not be in balance. Check out the ways to detect patterns below and talk to your endocrinologist, diabetes educator, or doctor.

☐ Once-a-day long-acting insulins like Lantus and Levemir last between nineteen and twenty-four hours for most people. To get better coverage, you may be better off to take these insulins twice a day. Check with your health care provider.

☐ Always check your blood sugar before you give yourself insulin.

☐ Eat snacks that combine a little protein and carbohydrate, like cheese and crackers or peanut butter and bread, to help keep your blood sugar level.

☐ Whether you have type 1 or type 2 diabetes, your insulin-to-carb ratio (how much insulin you need to cover carbohydrates) can be different at different times of day. For instance, you may need more insulin to cover the same amount of carbs in the morning when many people experience the Dawn Phenomenon (increase in blood sugar in the early morning hours), and you may need more or less insulin to cover the same amount of carbs in the afternoon and evening. Checking your blood sugar, and checking with your doctor, is the only way to know.

☐ I consider "routine" to be one of my most effective tools to maintain close to normal blood sugars. It may rob me of a little spontaneity, but eating and exercising similarly day to day helps me get more predictable blood sugars.

☐ Check out a great little invention—a cap with a digital readout, that works with any insulin pen, and tells you when you took your last injection. Available from Timesulin at timesulin.com. I have one and it's alerted me to a missed shot more than once.

☐ Switch out your boring black meter case for a small, brightly colored bag to carry your meter and supplies. You might just find it more inviting to check your blood sugar.

☐ Consider using a continuous glucose monitor (CGM). CGMs consist of a sensor you wear and an electronic receiver that shows you your blood sugar every few minutes and whether it's stable or going up or down (see "Do #34. Consider Whether an Insulin Pen, Pump, or Continuous Glucose Monitor Is for You").

☐ Have an A1C test two to four times a year and, you guessed it, discuss the result with your doctor to see if you need to make any changes to your current treatment plan.

More ways to detect patterns:

• Keep a record of your blood sugars that includes how much medicine you take, what you eat, what exercise you do, and when you're stressed. Bring this to your visit with your health care provider. Discuss what you're doing well when your blood sugars are in range, what might cause them not to be in range, and what to do about this.

• Use the Roche ACCU-CHEK® 360° View Tool to get a quick snapshot of how food, exercise, medications, stress and/or illness affect your blood sugar by checking your blood sugar three days in a row at seven different times of day: before breakfast, two hours after, before lunch, two hours after, before dinner, two hours after, and before bed. Download the paper tool here: accu-chek.com/us/data-management/360-view-printable-tool.html.

• Health care providers can use the Roche Diagnostic ACCU-CHEK® View Tool with their patients by downloading the tool here: accu-chekconnect.com/hcp/360-view-tool.html.

• Since God made seven days in a week, if you don't want to check more than once a day (I'm talking to type 2s now, type 1s need to check at least four times a day), you'll still get some valuable information by checking your blood sugar at a different time each day as well as writing down your medicine, meal, and activity. Monday, before breakfast, Tuesday, two hours after breakfast, Wednesday, before lunch, Thursday, two hours after lunch, Friday, before dinner, Saturday, two hours after dinner, and Sunday before bed. Share the results with your health care provider.

Do #24

Take a Peek at Your Feet

When was the last time you looked down there? At your feet, I mean! Sure, they're far away and sometimes hard to see and grab hold of, but when you have diabetes your feet need your attention—and an enormous amount of TLC (tender loving care).

Over time, high blood sugars, unfortunately, can cause circulation problems and decrease blood flow to your feet. One foot-related diabetes complication is peripheral arterial disease (PAD). PAD is generally associated with high cholesterol, high blood pressure, and insulin-resistance, all of which are common among people with type 2 diabetes. If you have PAD, you may feel cramping, pain, or tiredness in your legs, feet, and/or toes. You may see sores appear in these areas that take a long time to heal, and your feet may often feel cold. But be aware, 50 percent of people with PAD don't feel any symptoms. If you're over the age of fifty it's a good idea to get tested for PAD, since one in three people with diabetes over fifty has it.

High blood sugars can also cause another nerve-related foot complication called diabetic peripheral neuropathy (DPN). More than 20 percent of people with diabetes have DPN. Symptoms of DPN are tingling, burning or a throbbing sensation, shooting pain, and/or a deep itch in one or both of your feet and/or legs. Or, your feet may be numb to any sensation. Keeping your blood sugar well controlled is your best defense against PAD, DPN, and other foot complications.

If you do lose sensation in your feet, or if bacteria enters a crack in the skin on your feet, you can get a foot ulcer. A foot ulcer first appears as an open sore on your foot, and, if it is not treated, an infection can make its way into the tissue of your foot and then the bone. If you've lost feeling in your foot, you can walk around with a deep ulcer and not know it. This is often when a foot ulcer turns into a foot amputation.

While all this can leave you feeling downhearted, you can avoid many problems by having your feet checked regularly. My podiatrist, after helping so many people turn around a foot problem, summed it up this way: "Save your feet, it'll save your life, no joke!" Mind your tootsies. You want them healthy and well, and with you forever.

Quick-Starts

☐ **Wash your feet every day in warm (not hot) water to keep your skin smooth and supple, but don't soak your feet.** Soaking can dry out your skin and cause it to crack. Any cracks or openings in your skin can allow bacteria to enter.

☐ **If you've lost any sensation in your feet, wear shoes or hard-soled slippers in the house and don't go barefoot outside or on the beach.** This helps prevent getting a cut or burn. A women I interviewed told me she crossed her living room floor barefoot when a pizza delivery guy rang her doorbell by mistake. She stepped on a tack but didn't feel it. Then she got an infection and had to have her leg amputated. Always safeguard your feet.

Your Choice of More How-To's

☐ Here's a quick check for poor circulation: press your finger firmly into the skin of your foot for a few seconds. The tissue around your finger should lighten, as you've just pushed some of the blood away. Now, remove your finger. If the color takes longer than two seconds to return to the area, your circulation is likely less than normal.

☐ See a foot doctor, known as a podiatrist, every year for a full foot exam.

☐ Ask a podiatrist for an ankle brachial index test if you are over fifty, smoke, have high blood pressure or cholesterol, are overweight, or have a heart condition. This non-invasive, painless test is for PAD.

☐ If you see a podiatrist (foot doctor) every few months, have him trim your toenails. If not, trim them when they are softer right after washing your feet. Cutting straight across is generally recommended.

☐ Put a lotion on your feet after you wash them and they're still slightly damp. It will help hold in moisture and keep your skin from cracking. Dry in-between your toes, but don't put lotion there.

☐ For more information about DPN, check out the website diabetespainhelp.com.

☐ If you have pain in your feet or sores are slow to heal, a product called WarmFeet can help you visualize blood flowing to your feet. Patients who used WarmFeet in trials reduced their incidence of foot ulcers and healed faster. Learn more about WarmFeet at warmfeetkit.com.

☐ To be safe from infections, bypass getting a pedicure at the beauty or nail shop.

☐ If you get a blister, don't pop it! Put a band-aid over it and wear a looser, soft-padded pair of shoes, like sneakers.

☐ Buy shoes late in the afternoon when your feet will be slightly swollen. Break in new shoes by wearing them only an hour a day. I hate to say it gals, but high heels, open-toed shoes, and sandals can increase your risk of injury and infection.

☐ Always wear socks with your shoes. Wear cotton socks, or those that wick away moisture, and seamless socks if seams bother you. If you can't find seamless socks at your local department store, you can find them online by searching "seamless socks." If you wear knee-highs, make sure they're not tight or they may constrict your blood flow.

☐ Ask your doctor whether Medicare covers special shoes if you need them.

Examining your feet:

• After washing your feet, use your eyes and hands to examine each foot. Look and feel for redness, cuts, bruises, cracked skin, ingrown toenails, blisters, or any other sores. If you find anything suspicious, see your doctor right away.

• If you can't reach your feet to examine them, or your vision isn't sharp enough to do this yourself, ask a loved one or friend to help you. Using a mirror, with large handles to grip and hold it, may also work.

• Every time you see your regular doctor, take off your socks so he will check your feet.

Do #25

Get Thee to an Ophthalmologist or Optometrist

It doesn't matter if you can't spell these doctors' names, neither can I. An ophthalmologist and optometrist are both eye specialists. You should see either one at least once a year and here's why.

People with diabetes are more susceptible to eye disease because high blood sugars over time can damage the very small blood vessels behind your eye or cause them to burst. This is known as retinopathy and it's the most common diabetic eye disease. Burst blood vessels can leak fluid on the surface of your retina, the tissue at the back of your eye. At first you may have no symptoms of retinopathy, but as it gets worse you may see dark spots in your vision, reduced vision, and, at its worst, it can cause blindness. A dilated eye exam, which only an ophthalmologist and optometrist can perform (not your primary care doctor), can catch problems behind your eye when there's still time to stop further damage.

Macular edema is also a somewhat common complication of diabetes. This is when your retina swells due to blood vessels leaking fluid. As the condition develops, you may have blurred vision. You may also experience some vision loss and find it hard to focus clearly.

You also want your eye specialist to check for cataracts, a clouding of your eye's lens, which can develop at an earlier age in people with diabetes. After thirty-two years with diabetes, I had my first sign of eye trouble: a slow growing cataract. My ophthalmologist said there was nothing yet to do, we'd just keep an eye on it. And we have for the past seven years. It's growing so slowly, there's nothing to be done yet.

Also, have your eye doctor do a test for glaucoma, an increase in the fluid pressure inside the eye that can lead to optic nerve damage and vision loss. By seeing your eye specialist every year, or more if necessary, you'll have the best chance to keep seeing everything just like you should.

Quick-Starts

☐ **Pick up the phone and make an appointment with an eye specialist.** Have an exam every year, including a dilated eye test.

☐ **Work with your doctor to get your blood pressure under 130/80 mmHg if it's higher.** High blood pressure can cause damage to the blood vessels in the retina.

Your Choice of More How-To's

☐ Get an annual dilated eye exam from an ophthalmologist or optometrist. Bring sunglasses because when you leave your pupils will be larger and they will take in more light. I even have to draw the blinds in my home for a few hours after I get this test.

☐ See your eye doctor if you have blurry or double vision, dark or floating spots, pain or pressure in your eyes, or any other eye problem.

☐ Keep your blood sugar within your target range as best you can or your A1C (measurement of blood sugar over the past two to three months) under 6.5 or 7%.

☐ Don't smoke. Smoking narrows the small blood vessels in your eyes.

It's a full-time job you're <u>not</u> paid for:

Do #26

See Your Dentist Once or Twice a Year

When you were a wee thing and your mother said, "Don't put things in your mouth," she probably wasn't talking about dental instruments. At least I don't think so. Much as we might not like it, seeing the dentist once or twice a year is a must. It's very easy to have a gum or mouth infection and not yet know it. Like so many things—believe me I wish I didn't have to write this so often and you didn't have to read it—high blood sugar over time puts you at greater risk for gum disease and mouth infections.

Gum disease, also called periodontal disease, is a major cause of tooth loss in adults. High blood sugar can also slow your ability to heal from gum disease and mouth infections. And the longer you have the infection, the longer your blood sugar will be hard to control, which will slow your healing. A vicious circle indeed. Smoking is also a risk factor for gum disease, and when you have diabetes smoking can easily worsen gum and mouth problems and make your recovery slower.

Also, if you wear dentures, you need to have them, and your gums, checked at least once a year. Lastly, a word to the wise: diabetes specialist Dr. Richard Bernstein says if your blood sugars are higher than they usually are for no obvious reason, you may have a mouth infection.

Don't wait until something is "wrong" to see the dentist. Keep things from going wrong by seeing your dentist regularly.

Quick-Starts

☐ **Brush your teeth at least twice a day** and floss every day to help prevent gum disease.

☐ **Learn the signs of gum disease**—loose teeth and sore, red, or bleeding gums when you brush or floss. Wow, you've already aced this Quick-Start!

Your Choice of More How-To's

☐ See your dentist for a check up and cleaning every six months if you have your own teeth and every twelve months if you wear dentures.

☐ If your teeth are too tightly spaced for flossing, other cleaning tools like thin floss and water piks are available at your local pharmacy.

☐ If you treat a low blood sugar in the middle of the night, rinse out your mouth with water so the sugar doesn't stay on your teeth and gums.

☐ Choose a flavored toothpaste to make brushing more enjoyable. Personally I hate mint, the flavor of most toothpastes, but I'm a fan of Tom's fennel (tastes like licorice) and cinnamint (tastes like cinnamon) toothpastes. They also have orange-mango.

☐ Make sure your dentist knows you have diabetes when you see her so she will be extra thorough with your exam.

Do #27

Have a Sick Plan Before You Get Sick

Being sick can make your blood sugar rise higher than normal. How? Your body's under stress and releases stress hormones to help you fight being ill. But stress hormones also raise your blood sugar! A bad illness can cause very serious blood sugar problems. The important thing is to have a sick plan so you know how to take care of your diabetes when you're sick. You should create a sick plan with your doctor that will tell you how to handle your medicines and your food, how often to test your blood sugar, and other essential things he will want you to do.

You should also be aware of a very serious condition that affects mostly people with type 1 diabetes, and occasionally people with type 2. It's called diabetic ketoacidosis (DKA). DKA is a condition of high blood sugar that causes you to become dehydrated. This can lead to diabetic coma or even death. DKA happens when your body doesn't have enough insulin to use glucose for energy and begins to burn fat instead. A by-product of burning fat is ketones. Excess ketones can cause dangerous acidity in the blood. Be aware, you can also develop DKA if your blood sugar is low, especially if you've been vomiting.

The beginning symptoms of DKA are being thirsty, going to the bathroom often, high blood sugar, and high levels of ketones in your urine. The way to test for ketones is with a little kit you can buy (you don't need a prescription) at the drug store. The kit contains strips to do a simple urine test. Symptoms that come on next if you are in DKA include feeling tired, dry or flushed skin, vomiting or feeling nauseous, fruity breath (a young girl told me when she had DKA she smelled like roses), and trouble concentrating.

On rare occasions, people with type 2 diabetes can develop something like DKA called hyperglycemic hyperosmolar syndrome (HHS), hyperglycemic hyperosmolar non-ketotic syndrome (HHNS), or hyperglycemic hyperosmolar non-ketotic coma (HHNKC). Whew! Those are big words, but what you need to know is you may have one of these conditions if your blood sugar is extremely high, for instance over 500 mg/dl (27.7 mmol/l), and you're dehydrated. These can occur if you've been sick or had or have an infection. What you also need to know is any of these conditions can be life-threatening. If your blood sugar is really high and you're dehydrated or vomiting, call your doctor right away or get yourself to a hospital's emergency room.

For now, the best way to prevent a minor illness from becoming a major problem is to have a sick plan.

Quick-Starts

☐ **Continue to take your medicines. If you take insulin and you're sick, even if you're not eating much, continue to take your insulin and test your blood sugar often.** You may need to take even more insulin because stress hormones will raise your blood sugar.

☐ **Keep the phone numbers of your health care providers handy** and with your sick plan. Also have your doctor's contact information for the evening and on weekends.

Your Choice of More How-To's

☐ Work with your health care provider to create a plan to follow when you're sick. Make sure your plan includes:

- ○ when to call your doctor
- ○ how often to check your blood sugar
- ○ your blood sugar target zone
- ○ whether to check your urine for ketones
- ○ how to adjust your medicines and what to eat

☐ Talk to your doctor about getting the appropriate vaccinations to help prevent you from getting ill in the first place.

When you're sick:

- Take in plenty of fluids, about one cup every waking hour.
- Check your blood sugar every two to four hours and write down the number to keep track. If your blood sugar level rises above 240 mg/dl (13.3 mmol/l) and your doctor has told you to take extra insulin for high blood sugar levels, take the appropriate amount.
- If your blood sugar is over 250 mg/dl (13.8 mmol/l) while you're sick, have extra liquids that do not contain sugar, like water; diet drinks; decaffeinated tea; chicken, beef, or vegetable broth; sugar-free jello; and sugar-free ice popsicles.
- If your blood sugar is under 70 mg/dl (3.8 mmmol/l), have carbohydrates like fruit juice, ginger ale or regular soda, glucose tablets or gel, ice pops (not sugar free), jello (not sugar free), soups, and, if you can manage it, fruit, bread, crackers, rice, and/or cereal. Each of the following is one carbohydrate exchange: ½ cup apple or orange juice, ½ cup regular soft drink, 1 popsicle, 1 slice dry toast, 6 saltine crackers, 1/3 cup frozen yogurt, 1 cup plain yogurt, 1 cup Gatorade, ½ cup ice cream, ¼ cup sherbet and ½ cup regular jello.
- If you use insulin and your blood sugar is higher than 300 mg/dl (16.6 mmol/l), do a urine test to check for ketones every six hours. Also check for ketones if you use insulin and are vomiting or have abdominal pain. Call your doctor if you have ketones in your urine.

Call your doctor if:

- You've been sick or have had a fever for a couple of days and aren't getting better.
- You've been vomiting or have diarrhea for more than six hours.
- You have fruity breath and/or have moderate to large amounts of ketones in your urine.
- Your blood sugar level is lower than your target range and continues to stay there.
- Your blood sugar levels are higher than 240 mg/dl (13.3 mmol/l) even though you've taken extra insulin. Or if you take pills to control your blood sugar, it's over 240 mg/dl (13.3 mmol/l) before meals and stays there for more than twenty-four hours.
- You have symptoms that make you think you have a serious condition. For example, your chest hurts, you're having trouble breathing, your breath smells fruity, or your lips or tongue are dry and cracked.
- You aren't certain what to do to take care of yourself.

If you call your doctor, be ready to tell her:

- How long you've been sick.
- What medicines you've taken.
- Whether you can eat and keep food down.
- Whether you're losing weight.
- What your temperature, blood sugar, and urine ketone levels are.

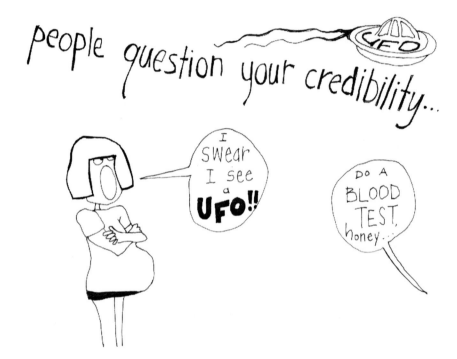

Do #28

Know What to Expect Before You're Expecting

When I got type 1 diabetes forty years ago, I was told I could never have children. The truth is I didn't, but not because I couldn't. Luckily, women are no longer being told they can't have children. Millions of women with type 1 and type 2 diabetes have successful pregnancies and deliver beautiful, healthy babies every day.

The best way to have a healthy pregnancy and deliver a healthy, bouncing baby is to plan ahead. Experts recommend that you work with your obstetrician and/or doctor at least three to six months before you get pregnant to make sure that your blood sugar, blood pressure, and cholesterol levels and your vascular (blood vessels) health are all in good control. Your doctor may also set specific goals like where your A1C (blood sugar average over the past two to three months) should be. Once you're pregnant, tight control of your blood sugar, especially in the first weeks of pregnancy, is the most effective way to guard against possible birth defects or troubles along the way.

During pregnancy, you can expect that your blood sugar levels will be erratic. They may be higher or lower than they normally are. You can expect to see your doctor often and have regular lab tests. Some women will need to check their blood sugar at home as many as ten times a day, including during the middle of the night. If you use insulin, you may have to take extra insulin during your pregnancy. Insulin requirements toward the end of pregnancy can be almost double. But once you deliver your baby, your insulin requirement will likely drop again. If you don't use insulin now, you may need to at some point during your pregnancy. If you have type 2 diabetes and you take pills for your blood sugar, you will likely be able to return to your pills after giving birth.

While this all may sound like a lot to do, here's the bottom line: take good care of yourself before and during pregnancy, and there's every reason to have a beautiful, healthy baby. Most women with diabetes do.

Quick-Starts

☐ **If you want to get pregnant, before you, oops, forget to put in your diaphragm,** set up an appointment with your obstetrician, endocrinologist, or family physician. You want to bring your blood sugar, blood pressure, cholesterol levels, and cardiovascular (heart) health to near normal levels before you get pregnant.

☐ **If you take ACE inhibitors or ARBs, check with your physician** whether you should stop taking them prior to getting pregnant.

Your Choice of More How-To's

☐ Try to reach a healthy weight, if you need to, before getting pregnant. Women who are overweight are at increased risk for cesarean deliveries and postoperative complications.

☐ If you smoke, stop. Period. No discussion. Your life and your baby's life depend on it.

☐ Have an A1C test every one to two months before getting pregnant.

☐ If you take pills to control your blood sugar, ask your physician whether you should continue taking them or switch to insulin prior to, and during, your pregnancy for better blood sugar control.

☐ If you feel you're in any risk, you may want to see a perinatologist. This is an obstetrician who specializes in high-risk pregnancies.

☐ Keep up your healthy eating and physical activity. They are just as important, if not more so, before and during pregnancy.

☐ You can connect with other women with diabetes who are pregnant, or have recently had babies, online at DiabetesSisters.org. Its founder, Brandy Barnes, created the site after searching for other women to talk with while she was pregnant herself.

Do #29

Seek Treatment if Your Sex Drive Has Taken the Off Ramp

Granted, fifty years of marriage may cool your engine, but so can high blood sugars. Erectile dysfunction (ED), the inability to get or maintain an erection, can affect as many as 50 percent of men who have diabetes within ten years of their diagnosis. High blood sugar and cardiovascular disease can damage the small and large blood vessels throughout the body, including the penis, limiting blood flow and making it difficult to have and maintain an erection. Diabetic neuropathy (a complication of diabetes that affects the nerves) can also contribute to difficulty having an erection.

Also, men who have diabetes are twice as likely to suffer from low testosterone, which can also cause ED. And the side effects from some medications may also cause ED. My friend Wil Dubois, diabetes treatment specialist and patient, points out that while some prescription medications for ED like Viagra, Cialis, and Levitra may help if what's blocking an erection is poor blood flow, they likely won't help if the problem is caused by nerve damage.

Diabetes can cause problems in the bedroom for women, too. Some women experience discomfort during sexual intercourse. Diabetes-related nerve damage can interfere with the vagina becoming lubricated when a woman is sexually aroused. This can cause discomfort or prevent a woman from feeling any sensation or reaching orgasm. Women with diabetes also tend to have more frequent vaginal infections and may experience vaginal itching or burning from prolonged high blood sugars. Every inch of you deserves your medical attention, including this area. Then it deserves someone else's attention, too, of course.

Quick-Starts

☐ **Sexual problems due to diabetes are treatable, so talk to your doctor.** He or she may recommend you see a specialist.

☐ **If you are male, have your testosterone level checked.** Low testosterone may cause problems other than ED, like decreased energy and strength. If this is the case, testosterone patches may be a treatment option.

Your Choice of More How-To's

☐ Devices like vacuum pumps, constriction rings, injections, penile suppositories, penile support sleeves, and implants may help make it easier to have and maintain an erection.

☐ Ask your doctor if any of the medications you're taking may be causing your erectile dysfunction. Diuretics, anti-depressants, and beta-blockers for blood pressure can cause ED.

☐ For women, prescription or over-the-counter vaginal lubricant creams like KY jelly may be effective for treating vaginal discomfort and dryness. Your health care provider may also have other options such as hormone suppositories and Viagra that some women use to enhance libido (sex drive). Also, check with your health care provider whether a medicine you're taking now may be affecting your libido.

☐ For women, antidepressants in the SSRI family, like Prozac, Zoloft, Celexa, and Paxil, can kill your libido and create difficulty getting aroused or reaching orgasm. They can also affect men but to a lesser degree. If you take one of these medications and are experiencing any sexual side effects, discuss your medication with your doctor.

☐ Limit your alcohol, reduce stress, and don't smoke. All of these factors can make erections harder to have and maintain for men and interfere with arousal for women.

☐ Keep your blood sugar well controlled. Blood sugar control may prevent the nerve and blood vessel damage that lead to erectile dysfunction and vaginal problems. It is truly your first line of defense.

Do #30

Give Up Smoking if You Smoke

We all know smoking isn't good for our health. But it's particularly unhealthy if you have diabetes. A recent study showed nicotine in cigarettes caused persistent elevated blood sugar levels and raised A1C levels (average blood sugar over the past two to three months) by as much as 34 percent!

Smoking also raises your LDL (lousy) cholesterol and your blood pressure, which can raise your risk for almost every diabetes complication, including heart attack and stroke, eye disease, vascular (blood vessel) disease, kidney disease, nerve damage, and foot problems. People with type 2 diabetes tend to already have high LDL and high blood pressure, so the last thing you want to do is raise it even higher. If you smoke, stop. If you don't smoke, don't start.

Quick-Starts

☐ **To cut down, buy a pack of cigarettes at a time, rather than a carton.** Carry only two or three cigarettes with you at any time.

☐ **Make three lists. The first is all the things you like and don't like about smoking.** The second is your reasons for wanting to quit. The third is what family and friends say they don't like about you smoking. Put the lists where you'll see them every day.

Your Choice of More How-To's

☐ Set a date to quit and tell your friends and family. Pick a time when your life is fairly calm and your stress levels are low.

☐ Throw away your cigarettes, matches, lighters and ashtrays.

☐ Use a nicotine patch or gum, inhaler, or spray, or discuss with your doctor the medicine Chantix. Chantix is a prescription medication that helps many people quit smoking.

☐ Ask your health care provider whether counseling, acupuncture, or hypnosis may help you quit.

Do #31

Keep Track of Your Medicines and Supplies

If you take more than a few medicines, it's easy to lose track of what you take, when you're supposed to take it, and when to re-order so you won't run out. It's also easy to lose track of how many supplies you have on hand (do you still have enough test strips, lancets, and pump supplies?) and where they all are. Managing your medicines and supplies is important but it shouldn't be a full-time job. If you get organized, you can set yourself up for success so you'll never (well, rarely) run out of what you need.

Quick-Starts

☐ **When you get a new prescription filled, mark on a calendar,** or set a reminder on your computer or phone, to re-order two weeks before you will run out.

☐ **Keep a list of all the medicines you take, including vitamins and supplements.** Next to each write down how many pills you take, the dose, and what time of day you take them. Keep a copy of the list in your wallet or purse.

Your Choice of More How-To's

☐ Get a pill box with the days of the week written on it, and on Sunday portion out your pills for the week. You can buy a pill box at your local pharmacy. Refer to the list you created to fill your pill box.

☐ Keep all your supplies in one place and where you can easily see what you have and when it's time to order more.

☐ Keep your medicines where you can see them and won't forget to take them, like on the kitchen counter (where I keep mine) or dining table. It's best not to keep your medicines in the bathroom (yeah, I know) where moisture from your shower or bath can spoil them.

☐ If you use a mail order pharmacy, see if they offer an automatic call when it's time to refill your medicines and/or supplies. Mine does, and it's a helpful reminder.

☐ Take your medicines around the same time of day, perhaps at the same time you do a daily activity. For instance, take a once-a-day pill before breakfast every day or before going to bed every night. Or create a way to remind yourself when it's time to take your medicine(s) like keeping a sticky note where you will see it or setting an alarm on your cell phone.

☐ Keep extra batteries in the house for your meter and insulin pump, if you use one.

☐ Keep an extra glucose meter in your office, school locker, car, or bag.

☐ Create a "go" bag for your supplies so you can easily grab them when you leave the house for the day. If you use insulin, always have glucose tablets and your meter in your "go" bag so you can check and treat a low blood sugar.

Do #32

Winterize Yourself Against the Flu

Each winter people get very sick and die unnecessarily from the flu. People with diabetes are three times more likely than people without diabetes to die from the flu or pneumonia. And each year 10,000–30,000 deaths among people with diabetes are associated with the flu or pneumonia.

For people with diabetes, the flu can be more than aches and pains. You may be ill for a longer time, or your flu may turn into pneumonia and you may have to go to the hospital for care. The flu is extra hard on people with diabetes since your immune system may be more vulnerable to a severe case of the flu. The stress to your body will play havoc with your blood sugars, which will then slow down your recovery (see "Do #27. Have a Sick Plan Before You Get Sick").

To increase your chances of not getting the flu, get a flu vaccine every year near the start of flu season (late September–early October) because it will take two weeks for the shot to become effective. While many people think flu shots can give you the flu, they can't. That said, after getting a flu shot you may feel a little achy or experience very mild flu-like symptoms for a day or two. That's your body's immune system gearing up to protect you against the real thing.

The Centers for Disease Control recommend the flu shot specifically for people with diabetes, including women with diabetes who are pregnant during flu season. Being pregnant can put you at risk for serious complications of the flu. Since the flu vaccine takes about two weeks to become fully effective, after you get yours take extra precautions not to be around people who may already have the flu.

Quick-Starts

☐ **To help reduce your chances of getting the flu,** wash your hands often with soap and water for at least twenty seconds or use a hand sanitizer. Do this even more often if you've been out in public—like riding the subway with a car full of coughers (yuck!)—or around anyone who's sick. Germs typically get spread when they land on you and you touch your eyes, nose, or mouth.

☐ **In the early fall, talk to your health care provider about you and your whole family getting a flu shot.** If everyone in your house gets the vaccine, you'll cut *your* chances down for catching the flu. What's better than protecting your loved ones, and yourself, at the same time?

Your Choice of More How-To's

☐ If your doctor says to get the flu vaccine, get it each year. Flu strains change every year.

☐ You can usually get a flu shot at a doctor's office, in clinics, pharmacies, and even some grocery stores. You can also call your local health department for dates, times, and places where flu vaccines are being given.

☐ Flu vaccines are available at little to no cost. Medicare Part B and many private insurance companies cover the flu shot.

Do #33

Know How to Inject if You Inject

Not so long ago, where on your body you injected made a difference as to how fast your medicine would go to work and how much of your medicine would actually get absorbed. With newer medicines and insulin analogs today, some think it doesn't make a difference where on your body you inject. Others still think injecting in your abdomen makes absorption more regular. There is one exception: if you use NPH insulin, you should inject in your thigh for best results.

You should also know injections you give yourself at home are nothing like what you might get at a doctor's office. The needle you use at home is very thin and short and only goes through the top layer of your skin. Most people say injections are painless or very rarely hurt. I agree.

Here are a few "rules-of-the-road" that will help you inject insulin or any other injectable diabetes medication.

Rule #1: Change your injection site so you don't inject in the same exact spot day after day. If you do, your body may build up scar tissue and it will be harder for the medicine you inject there to be absorbed. For each injection, use different spots on your abdomen, outer part of your thighs, buttocks, and the back of your arms.

Rule #2: We all know we're supposed to change our syringes and pen needles every injection, but does anyone, really? However, each time you inject, the needle dulls a little. So if an injection hurts or you're sawing through your skin, trust me, it's definitely been too long since you changed your needle! The American Diabetes Association recently said it's okay to re-use syringe needles if you don't have open wounds or live in a pig pen (the pig pen idea is admittedly mine), but never, ever share your needle. You don't share your toothbrush, do you? You should *absolutely* take your pen needle off the pen each time you use it. You can reuse the needle if you store it with its cover on and so it won't touch anything else. Taking the pen needle off after each shot keeps air bubbles from forming in the barrel. Air bubbles can prevent you from getting your full dose.

Rule #3: Using alcohol swabs before injecting was recommended in my early years with diabetes, but they are unnecessary and, in fact, tend to dry out your skin. Plus, using an alcohol swab can throw off results from some glucose meters.

Quick-Starts

☐ **If you use a vial and syringe, protect your vial from breaking with a Securitee Blanket at** securiteeblanket.com. This is a little cushioned tube you slip your vial into so it won't break if you drop it. So simple, so inexpensive, so valuable.

☐ **If you do find injections painful,** find out if you can get syringes that have thinner needles than what you're using now. If you can't, or you're already using the thinnest needle, ask your pharmacist to recommend a numbing cream.

Your Choice of More How-To's

☐ Keep insulin vials in the fridge until you're ready to use them. Then you can store them in the fridge or at room temperature.

☐ Keep insulin, Victoza, and Byetta pens in the fridge until you're ready to use them. Once you start using them, you must keep them at room temperature. In addition, do not store Victoza over 77 degrees Fahrenheit (25 Celsius) and Byetta over 86 degrees Fahrenheit (30 Celsius). Thermometer anyone?

☐ Cold medicine may sting. So if you just took your medicine out of the fridge, let it stand a few minutes or wrap your hands around it to warm it.

☐ Grab a pinch of skin before you inject to avoid the needle going into a muscle. You can skip the "pinch an inch" if using very short needles, 4mm or 5mm in length. I use BD's Ultra-Fine short 4mm Nano needle on my insulin pen and BD's Ultra-Fine, 31 gauge, short, half-unit syringes. The half unit markings help me make my dose more precise.

☐ Stay relaxed before an injection, inject quickly, and keep the angle of the needle going in and out straight.

☐ Inject in an area that you're not going to exercise. In other words, if you're going out for a run, don't inject in your thigh. The activity will increase the medicine's rate of absorption.

☐ If you have any problems with your vision or difficulty with your fingers, consider using Clickfine pen needles. Rather than needing to be screwed onto your pen, they simply click on with one motion and you can hear that they're attached. You'll find them at most major chain stores, drugstores and online at myclickfine.com.

☐ Talk to your health care provider about using an insulin pump. It's an investment of time to learn how to use the pump, and can be costly, but you'll only feel the prick of a needle every three days.

Preparing your dose when using a vial of insulin:

• If using a vial of intermediate or long-acting insulin that looks cloudy or milky-white, gently roll the bottle between your palms for fifteen seconds to mix it. Only cloudy-looking insulin needs to be rolled.

• Pull the plunger on your syringe back the same amount of units as your insulin dose.

• Remove the needle cap. Put the needle through the rubber stopper and push the plunger into the bottle.

• Turn the bottle upside down, leaving the needle in place.

• Pull the plunger down to measure your dose, using the black tip of the plunger to match the markings on the syringe. If you see air bubbles in the liquid, flick your finger against the barrel of the syringe to drive them up to the top and slowly push the plunger up to remove them. Then you may have to add a little more insulin. If that doesn't work, push the plunger up again fully to get the insulin back into the vial and withdraw it again. I once read, "three times a charm." In truth, you may not get rid of every teeny air bubble, and air bubbles in the syringe won't harm you. However, bigger ones can reduce the amount of insulin in the syringe.

• Pull the needle out of the bottle.

• Choose an injection site on your abdomen, thighs, buttocks, or back of your arms. Your abdomen, that fleshy part you probably think of as your stomach, stretches from the bottom of your ribs to your pubic line. Avoid injecting around your belly-button.

Injecting yourself with a syringe:

1. Use an appropriate needle length. While there are very short needles out today, if you have a thick layer of body fat where you'll inject, use a needle that's ½ inch long.
2. Hold the syringe like a pencil.
3. Pinch your skin and quickly insert the needle at a 90-degree angle.
4. Release the skin.
5. Push down on the plunger in a steady motion until the insulin has been injected. Pull the needle straight out. Sometimes you may see a small drop of blood or a bruise, which is quite normal.

Injecting yourself with a pen:

1. Use an appropriate needle length. While there are very short needles out today, if you have a thick layer of body fat where you'll inject, use a needle that's ½ inch long.

2. Prime an insulin pen (release any air bubbles in the insulin barrel) before each injection by dialing your dose to number "3." Hold the pen with needle pointing up. Tap the pen so any bubble goes up toward the needle. Push the injection button on the end of the pen. Repeat if you see an air bubble until it goes away. If this doesn't work, don't use the pen. Call the pen manufacturer. Likely they will send you a new pen. Air bubbles can occur with a new pen and they can also happen if you don't remove the pen needle after each use. If you use an injectable medicine other than insulin, you only need to prime the pen the first time you start the medication.

3. Dial up your dose using the dial at the end of the pen opposite the needle.

4. Quickly insert the needle into your body at a 90-degree angle.

5. Press the button at the end of your pen all the way down to release the medicine.

6. Hold the pen in your body for a count of ten seconds to make sure you get your full dose.

7. Pull the pen straight out. Sometimes you may see a small drop of blood or a bruise, which is quite normal.

Do #34

Consider Whether an Insulin Pen, Pump, or Continuous Glucose Monitor is for You

First let me say that if you have type 2 diabetes and your doctor is recommending insulin to manage your blood sugar, it doesn't mean you've failed or your diabetes has gotten worse. Insulin is one of the best medicines to control blood sugar. It's a natural hormone your body produces and almost half of those with type 2 diabetes will find themselves needing insulin as their beta cells (insulin-producing cells) wear out over time.

There are currently three ways to deliver insulin into your body: through a syringe, insulin pen, or insulin pump (or "patch" pump). A syringe and vial are pretty basic, you've seen them on medical shows a million times. People who take shots generally prefer insulin pens. They sort of look like a big fat pen with a small needle at one end and a plunger-like button at the other. Even though they're bigger than a syringe, most people who use them find them convenient to carry and more discrete than syringes. Many people also find insulin pens easier to use. You set your insulin dose with a "clicking system" you can hear and push the button to deliver the dose. In addition, most pens come with pre-filled insulin cartridges. So when the pen is empty, you just throw it away and start a new one. Now if only an insulin pen meant we could write "insulin" on our body and it would somehow magically get absorbed!

Insulin pumps deliver insulin most like a fully functioning pancreas (organ in your body where insulin is made) does. They deliver micro pulses—tiny amounts of insulin—every few minutes into your body. A pump can also give you a more accurate and much smaller dose of insulin than an insulin pen or syringe, and they work in "real time." If you decide to go exercise, for example, you can reduce, or stop, the amount of insulin your pump will deliver while you exercise. Pumps also provide many helpful features like a list of common foods with carb counts that you can customize for the foods you eat most often, dosing calculations, how much insulin you still have working in your body since your last bolus (meal time coverage), alarms, and more.

Insulin pumps deliver insulin into your body through a cannula (tiny flexible tube) attached to your skin. Most pumps also have a tube that goes from the pump to the cannula. Currently, there is one tubeless pump on the market called Omnipod, and there will soon be several more. There is also a very simple and small patch pump for people with type 2 diabetes called the V-Go. More and more companies are working ferociously to produce smaller pumps with more features, cooler looking screens, and greater connectivity between the pump and other diabetes devices. Currently the Animas Ping and Accu-Chek Combo System allow you to control your pump with a hand-held remote device that also contains a blood glucose meter. The T-slim pump just came out with a screen as cool and beautiful as an iPhone, and it fits in your pocket.

When I go out and talk to others with diabetes, they invariably ask me if I wear an insulin pump. I don't. To be honest, for me it's a trade off. A pump would probably give me slightly better control, but then be something extra I have to wear and deal with. My Virgo character already makes me extremely disciplined—I check my blood sugar five to ten times a day, take correction injections as needed, and am routine in my eating and exercise—so I'm able to keep my blood sugar in range most of the time.

Growing in popularity is the continuous glucose monitor (CGM). The advantage of a CGM is that it helps you see whether your blood sugar is stable, going up, or going down, and how quickly so you can better head off low and high blood sugar. A CGM consists of three parts: a sensor that slips under your skin and is held in place by adhesive, a transmitter that attaches to the sensor and relays your blood sugar reading, and the handheld receiver where you see your reading. Disadvantages of a CGM may be another device to wear and deal with, some don't yet provide the accuracy one might want, and their alarms sometimes go off inaccurately, and embarrassingly. By the way, you don't have to wear an insulin pump to use a CGM. And there's one pump/CGM system on the market right now—Medtronic's MiniMed Paradigm Real-Time Revel—in which the CGM wirelessly sends glucose information to the pump.

As a final note, a CGM checks the glucose in your interstitial fluid which lies just below the skin, not the actual glucose in your blood. So what you see on the display will be where your blood glucose was about ten minutes ago. So you should always double-check your blood sugar on your glucose meter if you think you should take more insulin to bring your blood sugar down or eat carbohydrate to bring your blood sugar up.

Quick-Starts

☐ **If you're interested, discuss these devices with your health care provider** and any friends you may know who use them. Since pumps and CGMs are costly, you will also want to find out if your health insurance covers them.

☐ **Ask if a diabetes educator will put a CGM on you for a week or two** and let you take a trial run. My friend, diabetes educator Gary Scheiner at Integrated Diabetes Services, offers this service and invites you to contact him, if interested, since he works nationwide. Check out integrateddiabetes.com or call his toll-free number: 877-735-3648.

Your Choice of More How-To's

☐ Ask your doctor about which insulin pen might be right for you.

☐ If you use more than one injectable medicine that comes in pen form, and they look somewhat similar, you may want to find a way to easily tell them apart. A friend of mine has a rubber band tied around one of her pens so she can easily feel the difference. You don't want to mix up your medicines.

☐ Check out the major insulin pumps online and see which one appeals to you. Manufacturers include Animas, Accu-Chek, Medtronic, Insulet, Tandem, and Nipro.

☐ Realize if you use a pump, it will be a learning curve. You will still be making bolus (meal time insulin) dosing decisions and will need to work very closely at first with a pump professional and your health care provider. You will also need to check your blood sugar at least four times a day and learn carbohydrate counting.

☐ Ask your endocrinologist or diabetes educator if you can wear a three-day sensor. The sensor tracks your blood sugar every five minutes. While you can't see your numbers until they get downloaded at your health care provider's office, you may get a feel for if you'd like to wear a CGM, and see trend information for what's working and what may be improved.

☐ Check out the different CGMs available online. Makers include DexCom and MiniMed (Paradigm and Guardian Real-Time).

☐ Make an appointment with a representative from a pump or CGM company if you are interested. They are very happy to show you their device and explain how it works.

☐ Some certified diabetes educators are also pump trainers and can help you learn how to use an insulin pump or continuous glucose monitor.

Do #35

Be Prepared for Hypoglycemia

Hypoglycemia, also known as "low blood sugar" or a "low," typically occurs when your blood sugar is less than 70 mg/dl (3.8 mmol/l). You may find your blood sugar that low, or lower, from time to time if you take a glucose (blood sugar) lowering medication like insulin or a sulfonylurea. Check the list of glucose lowering medications under "Your Choice of More How-To's."

Since hypoglycemia can be life-threatening, I want you to be knowledgeable about what it is and be as prepared as possible to prevent it and treat it if it occurs. What follows in this "Do" only pertains to you if you take a glucose lowering medication.

Going low can happen for several reasons, including:

• taking too much insulin or another medication that lowers your blood sugar

• taking too much medication for the amount of carbohydrates you eat

• taking your medicine and delaying or skipping your meal

• exercising more than you intended

- drinking alcohol

- becoming more insulin sensitive as you lose weight

- trying to maintain tight blood sugar control, which leaves you little cushion before going too low

Hypoglycemia can range from mild to moderate to severe. If you experience mild hypoglycemia, you may feel the following symptoms: shakiness, heart pounding, nausea, feeling cold or clammy, sweating, numbness or tingling in your fingertips or lips, and/or hunger. Moderate hypoglycemia, when your blood sugar falls below around 55 mg/dl (3 mmol/l), can bring on confusion or difficulty concentrating, mood changes like anger, irritability or anxiety, a lack of energy, poor coordination, fatigue, and slurred speech. Severe hypoglycemia, if your blood sugar falls below around 35 mg/dl (1.9 mmol/l), can cause convulsions, passing out, or even death. You may feel these symptoms even if your meter's numbers don't perfectly match the guideline. If you think your blood sugar is too low, and you have your meter and can check, then check. If you don't have your meter, treat it as if you are low just in case.

The recommended treatment for low blood sugar is to take 15–20 grams of fast-acting carbohydrate. The quickest carbohydrate to raise blood sugar is pure dextrose, which is found in glucose products that are available at your local drug store. Four glucose tablets or a glucose gel packet or glucose drink contain about 15 grams of glucose. Fast remedies to raise your blood sugar, other than glucose products, are half a glass of juice or regular soda, a glass of skim or low-fat milk, two tablespoons of honey, four or five saltine crackers, four teaspoons of sugar, or a handful of SweeTarts, Smarties, raisins, or jelly beans. Do not treat hypoglycemia with cake, candy, cookies, or any sweet that has fat in it. Fat slows down the absorption of carbohydrates. That's the reason to use skim or low-fat milk rather than whole milk.

Wait fifteen minutes after eating your carbohydrates and then check your blood sugar. If your blood sugar is still lower than 70 mg/dl (3.8 mmol/l), have another 15–20 grams of fast-acting carbohydrate and check again in fifteen minutes. Keep checking until your blood sugar is close to 100 mg/dl (5.5 mmol/l).

Be careful not to over-treat a low. Years ago, I'd often have a low blood sugar and, feeling ravenous and shaky, reach for anything and everything in sight to eat. I'd grab some bread and jam, cookies, fruit, *and* the last piece of pie in my fridge. Not long after I finished my little food-fest, my blood sugar was 300 mg/dl (16.6 mmol/l)! My last bit of advice: do wait until after you correct a low to put on your mascara, or you'll be wearing it all over your face—don't ask me how I know.

It's not always possible to prevent hypoglycemia, but you can do a number of things to safely treat it and help it occur less often.

Quick Starts

☐ **Carry a form of fast-acting carbohydrate with you at all times.** I have glucose tablets and SweeTarts or Smarties in all my jacket pockets (so does my husband) and my purses, and tiny SweeTarts rolls under my pillow. Some people carry the fruit candy Skittles. I carry some of my glucose tablets in a handy key chain case that costs under $5 and holds four glucose tabs. You can find it at quickfixkeychain.com/products.html.

☐ **Right now tell someone in your household what to do if your blood sugar is so low you pass out.** They should call 911 and give you an injection of glucagon if you have it and you've taught them how to do it. Glucagon is taken as an injection and raises your blood sugar if you can't swallow or are having seizures or become unconscious due to severe low blood sugar. You need a prescription to purchase a glucagon emergency kit, and you'll need to show someone how to mix up the ingredients and give you the shot, because you will not be able to do it yourself. Never ever have someone try to feed you or pour juice or soda down your throat. You can possibly choke.

Your Choice of More How-To's

☐ Ask your doctor if you're taking one of these medicines that lower blood sugar: glyburide (brand names DiaBeta, Glynase, and Micronase), glipizide (Glucotrol, Glucotrol XL), glimepiride (Amaryl), combination drugs that contain glyburide, glipizide, or glimepiride (such as Glucovance, Metaglip, Avandaryl, and Duetact), repaglinide (Prandin), and nateglinide (Starlix).

☐ Learn how to take the right amount of medicine for how many carbs you eat. Two systems for calculating this are the exchange system and carbohydrate counting. A diabetes educator or nurse can teach you these systems.

☐ Get a book like *The Calorie King: Calorie Fat & Carbohydrate Counter* that lists almost every food including foods from restaurants and fast-food chains to see how many carbohydrates they contain. I use it religiously. You can also use calorieking.com on your smartphone. The free app, "Carb Counting with Lenny," is an easy app for all ages, including children.

☐ As best you can, eat your meals and snacks at regular times and take your medications on time.

☐ Shift some carbohydrates from your meal plan to before you exercise in order to fuel your exercise and keep your blood sugar from dropping too low.

☐ Check and restock your fast-acting carbohydrate stash regularly, and always have some of your stash, like glucose tablets or a juice drink, in your car.

☐ Reduce the amount of insulin you take when you know you're going to be physically active. You'll have to judge based on how hard and how long you work out and by doing some research like checking your blood sugar before and after similar activity.

☐ If your blood sugar goes low often, talk to your health care provider about adjusting your treatment plan or medication.

☐ Consider wearing a continuous glucose monitor, which will alert you when your blood sugar is dropping.

☐ Keep a glucagon emergency kit in the house and buy a new kit every year since it expires in a year.

☐ Make family members, anyone you live with, coworkers, and friends aware of hypoglycemia and how to help you should you experience it.

Prevent hypoglycemia with blood sugar checks

- Always check your blood sugar:
  - ○ Before and after you exercise. If your blood sugar is 100 mg/dl (5.5 mmol/l) or less, bring it up to between 120 (6.6 mmol/l) and 180 (9.9 mmol/l), depending on how hard and how long you'll exercise. Strenuous activity can lower your blood sugar for as long as twelve to twenty-four hours afterward. So check your blood sugar a few hours after strenuous activity and a few hours after that to make sure your blood sugar stays within your target range.
  - ○ Before you drive and during your drive if you're driving a long distance. Pull over to a rest stop to check your blood sugar every few hours. Pull over to a rest stop if you feel you might be low. Correct your blood sugar, if necessary.
- Do frequent blood sugar checks:
  - ○ If you've had a number of "lows" within a few days or a week. When this happens, you may not feel the symptoms of a "low" until you begin having them less frequently.
  - ○ If you have "hypoglycemic unawareness" because you will not feel the symptoms of a "low".

• Get to know how much your blood sugar typically drops overnight by checking it on several nights just before you go to sleep and when you wake up in the morning. Based on how much your blood sugar drops overnight:

○ Keep it at a level before you go to sleep so it won't drop below 70 mg/dl (3.8 mmol/l). That may mean having a snack before you go to sleep. My blood sugar typically drops 30 points overnight. If I've had wine with dinner, the drop can be 50 points or more. I need to make sure my blood sugar is between 120 mg/dl (6.6 mmol/l) and 140 mg/dl (7.7 mmol/l) before bed to accommodate the drop. Since diabetes affects each of us differently, don't take my numbers for yours. You must know what *your* blood sugar does overnight.

○ Consider eating an Extend Bar before you go to sleep. Extend bars contain corn starch, which helps keep your blood sugar level for seven to nine hours. You can find them at extendbar.com, on Amazon.com, or near the pharmacy department in some chain stores like Walgreens, Walmart, Safeway, Wegman's, and others. I eat a few bites before bed on nights I've had some alcohol.

○ If you're a caregiver, or the parent of a child with diabetes, consider getting the mySentry Remote Glucose Monitor. It sits on your nightstand and displays someone's blood sugar from a continuous glucose monitor he or she is wearing in another room. It alarms when their blood sugar goes higher or lower than the target range numbers you set.

Do #36

Know if Weight-Loss Surgery is an Option for You

Weight-loss surgery, also called gastric bypass or bariatric surgery, has helped many people with type 2 diabetes both lose weight and lose their diabetes, so to speak. In fact, a study published in *The New England Journal of Medicine* reported that weight-loss surgery was more effective at treating obesity and diabetes than the conventional treatment of diet and exercise. Over a two year period, 75 percent of people who had gastric bypass had their diabetes symptoms go away (they had a fasting blood sugar of under 100 mg/dl or 5.5 mmol/l, and an A1C of less than 6.5% for at least one year). Comparatively, no patient in the non-surgical, medical lifestyle group had their diabetes symptoms disappear.

That said, a report by the Mayo Clinic that came out in June 2012 found that diabetes can return in up to 21 percent of patients who undergo gastric bypass surgery within three to five years. The strongest factor for diabetes recurring was patients having had diabetes longer than five years before their surgery.

Gastric bypass surgery is a minimally invasive procedure where a surgeon closes off most of the stomach, leaving only a small pouch to hold food. That pouch is about the size of an egg. This means you can only eat as much as that pouch can hold, obviously a very small amount at any one time. More than three out of four people with type 2 diabetes who undergo weight-loss surgery find their blood sugar returns to normal levels. Not after they lose weight, but within a few days of surgery. Scientists think a metabolic change causes glucose levels to return to normal.

Two other weight-loss procedures are gastric sleeve and gastric banding. In a gastric sleeve procedure, part of the stomach is removed and a small sleeve-shaped tube that limits food intake is left in place. In gastric banding, also called lap banding, a band is wrapped around the top portion of the stomach, again creating only a small pouch to hold food. Like gastric bypass, these procedures also help bring blood sugars back to normal range, although gastric bypass surgery seems to do so for greater numbers of people.

Many people with type 2 diabetes who undergo these procedures find they can reduce the amount of medicine(s) they take or stop taking their medication(s) altogether. If you have such a procedure, you'll have to take vitamins and supplements on an ongoing basis afterward (presumably for the rest of your life) because your body will be taking in fewer calories and nutrients.

Most patients who undergo these procedures do so without harm. Yet be aware, some people experience problems afterward such as nausea, vomiting, bloating, general weakness, and diarrhea. And in truth, even if one of these procedures works for you, your diabetes doesn't *really* go away, the symptoms do. If you put the weight back on, your diabetes will return.

Quick-Starts

☐ **If nothing else has worked for you to get to a healthy weight, talk to your doctor and see if you're a candidate for one of these procedures.** Typical candidates have a body mass index (BMI) over 30, sometimes over 35 (someone who is 5'8" tall and weighs 230 pounds has a BMI of 35), are between twenty and sixty-five years old, have tried to lose weight with diet and exercise many times and have failed, and have no history of alcohol, drug abuse, or a psychiatric disorder.

☐ **Check to see if your health insurance covers weight-loss surgery.**

Your Choice of More How-To's

☐ Familiarize yourself with the risks if you're considering having one of these procedures. You could experience a blood-flow blockage to the lung, a leak from the stomach after the procedure, a band that loosens, and what's called "dumping syndrome," which is gastric distress if food moves too quickly through the body.

☐ Make sure you're ready mentally to take on not only the procedure, but also how you will have to live afterward, which is eating very small amounts of food. Discuss this with your health care provider, a counselor, or someone who has had the procedure.

Do #37

Get Professional Help if You're Depressed

People with diabetes are two to three times more likely to experience depression than people without diabetes. It's not so surprising really. Diabetes is a lot to manage. It can be frustrating, overwhelming, confusing, and at times feel like a terrible burden. The trouble with depression is not only will it make you unhappy, but you won't have the energy or desire to take care of your diabetes.

How do you know if you're depressed? Here are some common symptoms: You find yourself unusually sad and it just won't go away. You struggle to get out of bed in the morning. You find it difficult to start, or do, anything. Your sleep pattern has changed. You don't feel like eating or you can't stop eating. Family and friends bring you no pleasure, and things that used to be fun aren't anymore. Or you may have suicidal thoughts.

If you're just feeling blue about your diabetes, or experiencing "burn-out," (that sense of "I've had enough!") doing one of the following things usually helps me. I talk about whatever's bothering me with my husband or a friend. I do something I like and so forget my troubles for awhile. And if I'm concerned about something in particular, I get more information. This helps me shake a bad mood and get back on track.

But if you think you're depressed, or a loved one is telling you they're concerned you may be depressed, seek help, or have someone do it for you. Don't let shame or embarrassment stop you from getting help.

Quick-Starts

☐ **If you can, maintain your regular exercise or take a short daily walk.** If you can walk in nature, even better. Nature calms us and exercise takes you out of your worries and releases endorphins—chemicals produced in the brain that make you feel better.

☐ **Listen to music that makes you feel good and smile inside.** Music lifts our mood, and makes us feel less stressed and more connected to the world.

Your Choice of More How-To's

☐ If any of the symptoms of depression sound like what you're experiencing, talk to your doctor. It's possible there's a physical reason for your feelings. If not, he may recommend medication and/or talking with a counselor, social worker, or therapist.

☐ Continue to take your medicine and follow your treatment plan. If this is difficult, discuss it with your health care provider.

☐ You can download a free app at findingoptimism.com for Apple and Windows computers and your iPhone or iPad, to track your mood, understand what affects your mental energy, and discover strategies to stay mentally healthy. Health care providers will find a version available to them to work with their patients who use the app.

☐ When something with your diabetes is getting you down, like mindless eating for instance, give it a person's name ("Tina," for example). See "Tina" as someone who is with you right now, but separate from you.

Think about times when "Tina" isn't with you at all. Can you create more of these times so that "Tina" is with you less often?

☐ See about joining an online diabetes community where you can share with others and feel less alone. Google "diabetes online community" and many will pop up.

☐ If you're a parent of a child with type 1 diabetes, check out the website Children with Diabetes at childrenwithdiabetes.com. It's a community for families and type 1 adults, and it's chock-a-block with resources.

☐ Check out the Behavioral Diabetes Institute (BDI) at behavioraldiabetesinstitute.org, which offers information and classes dealing with depression and managing the emotions of diabetes. If you're just feeling burned out, check out founder of BDI, Bill Polonsky's classic book, *Diabetes Burn Out*.

☐ If you're a medical professional and want to check your patients' diabetes distress, you can use the "Diabetes Distress Scale" developed by psychologist and CDE Bill Polonsky at familymedicine.medschool. ucsf.edu/pdf/bdrg/scales/DDS_all.pdf.

☐ Check to see if there's a support group in your community or talk with someone else who has diabetes.

☐ If you can, volunteer in your community. Helping others is a great way to take your mind off your own problems.

Do #38

Schedule Doctor Visits Around Your Birthday

Here's a tip to make sure you see all your doctors *at least* once a year. That might include a podiatrist (foot doctor), ophthalmologist or optometrist (eye doctors), endocrinologist (diabetes specialist), family doctor, diabetes educator or nurse, dentist, dietitian, as well as any other specialist you see (or should see) on at least a yearly basis. Make all your appointments in your birthday month. That way you won't forget. Of course, if your birthday is in winter, and you live in North Dakota, hmmm…you might want to schedule your appointments around the fourth of July. The point is by seeing your health care providers on a regular basis, you can often catch a diabetes complication early and stop or slow its progress. In my book, that's the best birthday present there could be.

Quick-Starts

☐ **Pull out your calendar, paper, cell phone, whatever you use, and write a reminder** to yourself to schedule your doctor visits starting a few weeks before your birthday or chosen month.

☐ **If you can book next year's appointment when you leave your doctor, do it.**

Your Choice of More How-To's

☐ If you can't get an appointment in your birthday or chosen month take the next closest appointment.

☐ For those doctors you should see more often (every three or six months), use your birthday or chosen month as a starting point and count out from there.

Any diabetic worth their salt has
two meters:

one for you

...and one
for
your doctor

Do #39

Bring Your Doctor These Questions

You'll get the most out of your doctor visit if you bring questions and you're honest and open. As for the latter part, share any concerns you have about aches or pains, family history, bodily changes from the last visit, or physical sensations you've noticed. Something diabetes-related may be happening and it will pay to catch it early. If you're just feeling blue, share that too.

Don't let fears, worries, embarrassment or guilt stop you from talking frankly with your doctor. She's not there to judge you, but to help you. If you haven't been doing a stellar job managing your diabetes—if you slid on doing your blood sugar checks for days or weeks, fell off your eating plan more days than you care to count, forgot to take your meds a few days last week, even if you feel like you are the laziest, most shameful person walking the Earth—don't lie. (That cartoon with the two meters is just that—a cartoon we can all identify with, but it's meant to make you laugh, not do!) Trust me, you aren't the only one your doc's going to see that day who didn't turn in a picture-perfect performance.

Dr. David Agus is an international leader for new approaches in personalized health care and professor of medicine at the University of Southern California, Keck School of Medicine. He says the knowledge *you* carry about yourself is more essential to your wellness than your doctor's knowledge. So hiding your several trips to the bathroom during the night, or the tingling you've noticed in your foot since your last visit, can do you harm. Dr. Agus is so emphatic that he also says if you feel you can't talk to your doctor, find another doctor!

You'll also get more out of your visit if you ask your doctor questions that will help you understand your condition better and what to do next. A number of recommended questions follow the "How-To's" below. Don't feel like you're being disrespectful by asking your doctor questions. Any good doctor will appreciate that you want to be involved in your care. Also, make sure you understand the answers to your questions. If you don't, ask your doctor to explain what they mean. The more you "show up" for your office visit, the better you'll be able to take care of yourself after you leave.

Quick-Starts

☐ **Bring a friend or loved one with you.** They can help be a second set of eyes and ears.

☐ **Bring paper and pen to write down your doctor's answers.**

Your Choice of More How-To's

☐ Think about anything you're concerned about before your office visit, write it down, and bring it to your health care provider to discuss. We tend to forget things when we're nervous or in the short amount of time we have with our doctor.

☐ While talking with your doctor, mention what comes to mind even if you think it might be unimportant. This might be just the information your doctor needs to know to help you.

☐ If your doctor has prescribed a new medicine, make sure you understand what it's for, when to take it, how much to take, what to do if you forget to take it, and if there are any side effects.

☐ If your doctor gives you any instructions, write them down before you leave his office so you'll know what to do when you get home.

Questions to help you get the most out of your visit:

1. "How am I doing?"
2. If you've recently had any lab work or tests, ask:
    a. "What were the results of my lab tests?"
    b. "What do they mean?"
    c. "What should I do to improve my numbers?"
    d. "Can I have a copy of my results?"
3. "Is it time for me to have an A1C test?" (An A1C test tells you your blood sugar average over the past two to three months. You should have the test two to four times a year.)
4. "How often should I check my blood sugar?" or, "Can we discuss the blood sugar results I brought?"
5. "What's going well so far?" and "What am I doing well?"
6. If you need help, "Can you help me with my meal and physical activity plans?"
7. "What should I focus on now?"
8. "Who else should I see for my diabetes care?"
9. "Would you please examine my feet and take my blood pressure?"

Do #40

Add a Medical Alert Bracelet to Your Jewelry Collection

I'm going to give you a $15 tip that can save your life: wear a medical alert piece of jewelry that says you have diabetes. If you're in an accident or your blood sugar drops so low that you can't treat it, you want a paramedic or a passer-by to know you have diabetes. That way you have a much better chance of getting medical attention and not thrown in the slammer. Severe low blood sugar can make you look like you're drunk: your thoughts are muddled, you may slur your words, you may become irrational or aggressive, or you may shake or have a seizure.

I don't know why most doctors don't tell their patients to wear medical alert jewelry, but I'm telling you. As someone who travels frequently, and often travels alone, my medical alert bracelet is just part of the jewelry I wear, along with my tiara of course.

Quick-Starts

☐ **Pick up a simple and inexpensive medical alert bracelet** at your local pharmacy.

☐ **Right now while you're searching for just the right piece of medical alert jewelry,** put an emergency card in your wallet with your medical information. You can create one at medids.com/free-id.php. You can also create one in no time by taking a small piece of paper that will fit in your wallet and writing down your name, date of birth, address, emergency contacts, doctor's name and phone number, your conditions, and the medicines you take.

Your Choice of More How-To's

☐ Make sure you can fit the most important information on your medical alert jewelry like your name, that you have diabetes, any other condition you may have, and an emergency phone number.

☐ Protect yourself while driving with any of several inexpensive medical alert items from Medical Awareness Decal at www.dadinnovations.com/products.html. Choose from a diabetic driver license plate frame, inside and outside window decals, and a "Diabetic Driver" key chain.

Websites for medic alert jewelry:

• Choose from a wide selection of bracelets, necklaces, charms, dog tags, and bag-tags from American Medical ID at americanmedical-id.com or Medic Alert Foundation at www.medicalert.org. Medic Alert Foundation also offers a free registry where you can store your health information online.

• You can find fun and fashionable medical alert jewelry for adults and children on many websites. Here are three: Sticky Jewelry, stickyj.com/medical-emergency.html, Lauren's Hope, laurenshope.com, and Children with Diabetes at childrenwithdiabetes.com/d_06_700.htm. Just make sure your medical alert jewelry doesn't look *too much* like jewelry or others may overlook it. Having the emergency symbol in red helps.

• If you'd like something a little sportier, check out Road ID at www.roadid.com. They make alert wristbands and other apparel.

• Wrap a small medical alert symbol around your watchband. It's available from MediBand at www.id-technology.com.

Shared Learning

Since we learn from each other, here are some personal "How-To's" from people living with diabetes:

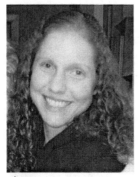

Alyssa

I work really hard to get that first blood sugar reading of the day in range. It sets the tone physically and mentally for the rest of the day. I often check in the middle of the night if I think something might go awry so I can catch it before the start of the day. I also keep Smarties and Starbursts everywhere—friends' houses, offices, in the car, in my purse, by my nightstand (where there's a book light so I don't have to turn on a bright light), and in the kitchen—so I don't have to worry about where I might be low and what to do.

> — **Alyssa Rosenzweig**
> 24 years old, living with diabetes 14 years.

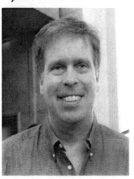

Seth

Now I always have extra pump supplies on hand and an unexpired bottle of insulin and syringes in a known, easy to find place for emergencies. When my pump accidentally got disconnected, I was unprepared. Even though I keep a bottle of rapid acting insulin and syringes in my office, it took me more than a panicky hour to find them!

> — **Seth Bernstein**
> 51 years old, living with diabetes 25 years.

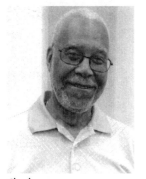

Charles

I always carry a kit with me that contains my insulin, needles, glucose tablets, test strips, lancets, meter, and alcohol swabs. This is an extension of my body. I never leave home without it.

> — **Charles Wiggins, Jr.**
> 79 years old, living with diabetes 9 years.

Your Quick-Start "Do" Sheet

Use this worksheet to help you accomplish any Medical "Do" in a way that works best for you.

The "Do" I will do is:

_____

_____

_____

Why it's important to me to do this:

_____

_____

_____

My "How-To" is/are:

_____

_____

_____

When I will begin:

_____

_____

_____

How often I will do this:

_____

_____

_____

Where I will do this:

_____

_____

_____

Who can support me:

_____

_____

_____

What can stop me:

_____

_____

_____

What I will do about that:

_____

_____

_____

What was successful and how I can keep doing it:

_____

_____

_____

Fitness Do's

Keeping fit makes everything work better.
Start with very small steps, like turning this page.

To keep yourself safe, talk to your health care provider
before beginning a fitness routine. He or she may recommend
a heart health assessment before you begin.

Walk-a-thons...

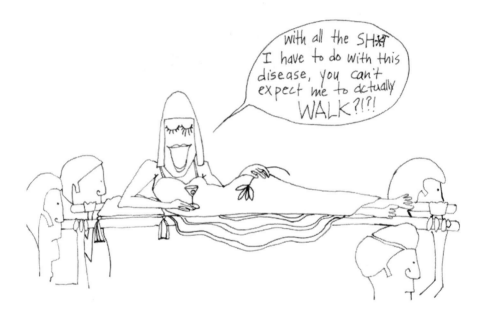

Do #41

Understand that Exercise is Medicine

That's a bold statement, but it's true. Just look at all the body benefits of exercise, or regular physical activity, without taking any medication. Exercise helps lower your blood sugar, blood pressure, LDL (lousy) cholesterol, and A1C. It can even keep your blood sugar lower hours after you exercise. That's because exercise increases your sensitivity to insulin. And people with type 2 diabetes (and some with type 1 diabetes) are resistant to insulin, meaning their bodies don't use insulin effectively.

Physical activity improves circulation, lowers your risk for heart disease and stroke, and builds bone and muscle. It increases feel-good hormones and boosts your brain power, leaving you less likely to suffer from dementia. It helps your body metabolize stress hormones, it helps you sleep better, and it burns calories to lower or maintain your weight. Just stretching helps you stay flexible, prevents stiffness, and can give your joints more range of motion. Exercise can help improve your balance to help you stay steady on your feet. Trust me, if exercise came in a pill we'd all be taking it!

Ideally, a well-rounded exercise program includes cardio work, strength training, and stretching. Cardio gets your heart rate up for an extended period of time, strengthens your heart and lungs, burns calories, and lowers body fat. Strength training keeps your bones strong and prevents you from losing muscle mass. Stretching keeps you flexible and less susceptible to joint pain.

You don't have to run a marathon, swim an ocean, bike cross country, or train for a triathlon to be fit or healthy. Although if you do—great! Just know that physical activity is good medicine and that doing it will help protect you throughout your lifetime.

Quick-Starts

☐ **Warm up before exercise.** Take a five minute walk or do some gentle stretching, or both. Then cool down with the same to help prevent injuries.

☐ **Drink water before and after activity and during activity** if it's of high intensity.

Your Choice of More How-To's

☐ Participate in the Big Blue Test this November 14th at bigbluetest.org, or just learn from this annual event. Thousands of people with diabetes have shown that doing just fourteen minutes of physical activity, on average, lowers blood sugar about twenty points.

☐ Ask your doctor to write you a prescription for physical activity, and then fill it.

☐ If you haven't been moving much, start off with a daily ten to fifteen minute walk. Increase your walk by five to ten minutes each week.

☐ Listen to your body and trust your intuition to tell you when you're overdoing it. Overdoing is an easy way to injure yourself. For moderate activity, you should be able to carry on a conversation while exercising.

☐ Take some small steps for improving your balance: walk backward or sideways, walk heel to toe in a straight line, stand on one foot, stand up from a seated position.

☐ Yoga and pilates, as well as stretches you do in a class or just simple stretches at home, are great ways to increase your flexibility. When doing stretches, don't bounce but hold each stretch for about thirty seconds and then switch sides. For a slide show of simple stretches from the Mayo clinic go to www.mayoclinic.com/health/stretching/SM00043.

☐ If you're athletic and ambitious, Dr. Oz offers an invigorating seven-minute video workout. It's a combination of yoga and stretching. I tried and discovered it was hard for me. But you can check it out at doctoroz.com/videos/dr-ozs-seven-minute-workout.

How to stay blood-sugar safe:

• Always check your blood sugar before and after exercise to learn your body's response to exercise. If you take insulin or a blood sugar lowering pill that puts you at risk for low blood sugar (ask your doctor or pharmacist if this means you), exercise may drop your blood sugar too low (see "Do #29 Be Prepared for Hypoglycemia"). Exercise will affect your blood sugar depending upon how long you are active and how hard you are working. If you are at risk for low blood sugar, and your blood sugar is under 100 mg/dl (5.5 mmol/l) before you start any physical activity, eat some fruit or crackers or have a glass of milk or juice to raise it. Then check your blood sugar after exercising. You want it to be in or near your target range.

• According to the American Diabetes Association (ADA), depending on the duration and intensity of exercise, you can continue to burn glucose (blood sugar) up to twenty-four hours after you exercise. The ADA recommends checking your blood sugar every forty-five minutes after a hard workout to see whether your blood sugar is going down, going up, or leveling off. If it is going down, eat some carbohydrate and keep checking until it levels off.

• If you have type 1 diabetes and your blood sugar is high and you want to exercise, first test to see if you have ketones. Ketones are dangerous fatty acids that build up in the blood when you don't have enough insulin in your system. You test for ketones in your urine with a ketone kit you buy at the pharmacy. If you have ketones, exercise can raise your blood sugar and produce even more ketones! Exercise after you are no longer producing ketones. The truth is, you probably aren't going to feel well enough to exercise before then anyway. If your blood sugar is "high" (above 250–300mg/dl or 13.8–16.6 mmol/l) but you are not producing ketones, exercise is likely safe and you can expect it to lower your blood sugar.

• If you take insulin or a glucose lowering drug, always carry some fast-acting carbohydrate with you, like glucose tablets, SweeTarts, Smarties, or juice.

• Wear a medical ID so people know you have diabetes in case your blood sugar goes too low or you have an accident or injury. If not, they may think you've been drinking because symptoms of low blood sugar can look like being drunk.

Do #42

Realize Exercise Doesn't Need a Special Outfit

Exercise doesn't just take place in a high-priced gym surrounded by rail-thin or muscle-bound model types who can lift 100 pounds, or do high-impact aerobics without breaking a sweat. In fact, lots of exercise takes place when you're not even aware you're exercising. For instance, you're exercising when you're vacuuming the dust bunnies out from underneath the bed, trimming your rose bushes, mowing the lawn, dancing to your favorite tune when nobody's looking, or walking miles to the mall cursing under your breath because you couldn't get a closer parking space.

Moving more throughout the day burns calories and it doesn't matter where it happens, if you paid for it, or whether you're wearing the latest tiger-striped leotard or jersey. And recent research tells us that moving throughout the day is as important, if not more important, than a dedicated half hour or hour of activity.

Quick-Starts

☐ **If walking is your muse, get a pair of shoes or sneakers** that support and truly fit your feet. A good pair of shoes will "take a load off" your joints and lower back, which will reduce overall inflammation.

☐ **Find small opportunities to move a little more throughout the day.** If you sit at a desk at work, get up every forty-five minutes or hour and take a five minute stroll. I walk up the two flights of stairs to my apartment unless I'm carrying three suitcases, two bags of groceries, and a sofa, which then of course makes it difficult.

Your Choice of More How-To's

☐ While exercise doesn't require a special outfit, sometimes a beautifully sequined leotard or a high tech moisture-wicking jersey in your favorite color may motivate you.

☐ Wear casual dress shoes at work or in more formal settings made by a running or walking shoe company. These keep you comfortable all day, and may inspire you to climb that flight of stairs instead of taking the elevator.

☐ Think about investing in a standing desk. Just like it sounds, you stand at this desk to do your work. Many say the endless hours we spend sitting are changing our metabolism for the worse and causing us to be less healthy. Standing, you'll burn more calories and may find you are more alert and have more energy.

☐ If you have a hobby that involves movement, do more of it, or try out something you've wanted to do like fishing, golf, gardening, hiking, trapezing or my curiosity, rock climbing.

☐ Make Sundays a day in the park with your family and you be the one burning calories by running after the frisbee when it falls in the baseball field.

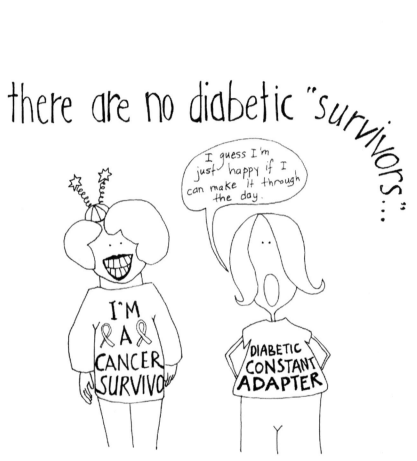

Do #43

Find an Activity that Fits You

Whether you'd like to just add a little more physical activity to your day or start a bona-fide exercise program, here's a "golden rule"—pick something you'll enjoy. If you don't enjoy it, trust me, you won't be doing it for long. If you don't currently have a physical fitness regimen, think about ways in which you like to move your body. Do you find yourself swinging your hips when you hear snappy salsa music? If so, consider taking a dance or aerobics class that has great music. Maybe you love Kung Fu movies. Martial arts anyone? One man told me he found love—and an easy way to get exercise—when he got a dog! Now he takes at least three walks a day.

If you're going to try a new activity, also try on a new attitude: think of it as an "experiment." Trying things out as experiments means you can't fail. When you experiment, you're playing a "win-learn" game, not a "win-lose" game!

If you have a limitation, or find you're just not that steady on your feet, that doesn't let you off the hook. There are many ways in which you can be active. Most YMCAs have pools, and moving in water is a great way to exercise without stressing your bones or muscles. Many senior centers offer classes like low-impact aerobics or chair dancing. I saw a dozen people in chairs doing upper body movements to music at a health fair, and they were having fun and working their butts off! There's no reason not to move, and many good reasons to find something that will move you.

Quick-Starts

☐ **Take the first step to learn more about an activity you've always wanted to try.** Stop at the gym for a booklet, search for the activity online, talk to a friend who does it.

☐ **If you have a limitation, consult your doctor.** Ask him for a referral to an exercise physiologist or physical therapist who can recommend exercises that will work for you.

Your Choice of More How-To's

☐ Consider a few sessions with a personal trainer. Trainers come to your home or you can meet them at a gym. They'll design a program tailored just for you and help you move so you don't injure yourself.

☐ If you have neuropathy (nerve damage caused by diabetes), which can make walking difficult, try short periods of walking. Or use a stationary bike, row, swim, or take a chair exercise class. A woman told me she gets her walk at the supermarket using the grocery cart for support.

☐ Check out these simple exercise videos with fitness trainer, Kim Lyons, on the *Take the Next Step* website, diabetespainhelp.com/nerve-pain-and-diabetes-management.aspx. I know Kim and she is passionate about helping people who have pain in their feet, move.

☐ Many websites can guide you on your fitness journey with information, resources, videos, and online tracking tools. Here are a few:

○ The American Diabetes Association website has a whole fitness segment that can get you started. Go to www.diabetes.org/food-and-fitness/fitness/?loc=DropDownFF-fitness.

○ Fit4D at fit4d.com has online coaches who will work with you as your guides and personal cheering squad.

○ dLife at dlife.com/diabetes-food-and-fitness has plenty of good information, as do Shape magazine's website, shape.com/fitness, and fitness.com.

○ Insulindependence at insulindependence.org offers positive and challenging "real world" adventure experiences and programs. With a group you can overcome fears, stretch your capabilities, and learn "keep-going" strategies to help in your daily management.

☐ For ten minutes a day, close your eyes and see yourself in pleasant surroundings. See your body as strong, flexible, and beautiful. Don't try to fix anything about your body, just enjoy the picture of a strong, healthy you. Practice often and in time your physical condition will begin to move closer to your mental picture.

☐ If you have retinopathy (a diabetes complication where the blood vessels at the back of your eye become damaged), weight lifting can make your condition worse. Discuss any weight-bearing exercises with your doctor.

Do #44

Embrace Regularity: Be Active Five Days a Week

Thirty minutes of low to moderate-intensity aerobic activity (using the same muscles rhythmically like when you walk, jog, swim, or in an aerobics class) five days a week is the fitness recommendation for all Americans. It's also the recommendation from the American Diabetes Association (ADA) for people with diabetes. But before you say, "I can't!" the ADA says you can spread those 150 minutes of activity over a week, any way you chose, as long as you don't go more than two days without any physical activity. And, if thirty minutes of activity is hard to fit into your day in one chunk, you'll get as much benefit from three brief ten minute spurts of movement.

While being active most days of the week is healthy, being a weekend athlete—getting very little activity during the week and then going all out on the weekends—is not. You're more likely to pull a muscle or get an injury, and you're more susceptible to a heart attack or stroke by only working out on the weekends. Make moving a daily habit and move throughout the day as best you can. Once it's a regular part of your schedule, you'll wonder how you ever did without it.

Quick-Starts

☐ **Squeeze in a few bursts of activity today.** Walk around your office, take the stairs, park your car farther away, throw a few hoops, do some bicep curls, or walk through your house like my mom does.

☐ **Lay out your workout clothes the night before.** When you wake, you'll have a reminder to work out and extra motivation.

Your Choice of More How-To's

☐ Always begin with a warm up of a short walk or some stretches and then do the same after your exercise to cool down.

☐ Break up boredom by mixing up activities: walk a few days a week, swim and bike once a week, hit the roller-rink or bowl once a month.

☐ If you have proliferative retinopathy (broken blood vessels at the back of your eye) or uncontrolled high blood pressure, make sure you get the okay from your doctor before starting any new exercise routine.

☐ Think whether a device can help you. I use a pedometer (it counts your steps) from Omron called "Pocket Pedometer." It's flat and it slips into, and sits inside, my pocket when I go out to walk.

☐ For more feedback, try a Fitbit, available at fitbit.com. It tracks your steps, stairs climbed, calories burned, workouts, and food logs. My husband got one and began offering to take out the garbage so he could get more exercise walking up and down the stairs!

☐ Train for a walk where you also do good like the American Diabetes Association or JDRF walks or runs.

☐ If you need an extra incentive, not to sound crass, but how about cash? Check out Gympact at gym-pact.com.

Do #45

Start with a Single Step and Aim for 10,000 a Day

Maybe you've heard this recommendation: walk 10,000 steps a day for general fitness. In 1996, in an effort to battle excessive weight and obesity, the US Surgeon General called for Americans to get thirty minutes of moderately intense activity in addition to their normal daily activities. That translates into walking 10,000 steps, or a distance of five miles, a day. That's a great goal, but likely a big one for most people. But success is in the details: approach big goals with small steps.

I power walk an hour a day. Six days a week, I step out of my building, walk two streets to a large park near where I live, and walk around the park. By time I'm back home wiping the sweat off my brow (and just about everything else), an hour has passed and I've hoofed 7,210 steps. Running errands and chasing after things I lose in the house usually adds another few thousand steps.

But I didn't start out power walking around the park. I started out taking short walks and then increased my time and steps as it became easier. You may see health benefits from walking just 1,500 or 2,000 steps. And don't underestimate the power of walking. When you feel physically strong, you become emotionally strong. And just walking can do that for you.

Quick-Starts

☐ **Walk in a good pair of sneakers, running or walking shoes.** Be sure they fit your feet and are well-padded, cushioned, and supportive. If your shoe store has a pedorthist (a health care professional who specializes in supportive shoes and inserts), he or she can help you pick a well-designed, best-for-you pair of shoes.

☐ **Wear a pedometer, a small instrument that counts how many steps you take.** Omron produces very reliable and easy-to-use quality pedometers. Seeing how many steps you're taking can motivate you to take a few hundred more. It can also be truth-telling when you see how few steps you're taking.

Your Choice of More How-To's

☐ If you have concerns about your ankles, knees, or hips, discuss a walking plan with your doctor before beginning.

☐ When you see your doctor or podiatrist (foot doctor), ask for a shoe recommendation.

☐ If gadgets really get your juices flowing, you might enjoy walking with a Fitbit Ultra (see fitbit.com). Not only does it track your steps like a pedometer, but it can track the number of floors you've climbed, measure your sleep activity, and even display motivational phrases. The device syncs your data wirelessly through a USB dock plugged into your computer, and you only have to charge the battery once a week.

To start a walking program:

• Wear a pedometer every day for two weeks and walk just as you do now. At the end of each day, jot down how many steps you took.

• At the end of two weeks, see how many steps you took each day. Take the highest number of steps you did and make that your daily walk goal.

• Walk your goal number of steps for the next two weeks.

• Every two weeks, add 500 steps. Continue until you reach 10,000 steps a day.

• If you need to slow this down and take fewer steps, do so.

Do #46

Plan To Be the Next
"Biggest Winner"

Maybe you've seen the enormously popular weight-loss TV show, *The Biggest Loser*. A number of very overweight contestants are brought to a ranch where their meals are prepared and they exercise for endless hours a day. Most, if not all, of the contestants do lose weight, but it's a very controlled environment and they have a team of experts to guide and help them. Let's face it, you probably don't have someone cooking all your meals or yelling at you to keep exercising when you feel like you can barely stand up.

That said, we can't deny that 68 percent of Americans are overweight or obese, including one in three children. Or that many people with type 1 diabetes and about three-fourths of people with type 2 diabetes are overweight or obese. And we can't deny that eating healthy, maintaining a normal weight, and getting physical activity are the most important things to do, along with taking your medicines, to manage diabetes.

So what role does exercise play in losing weight? Let's take a look: If you walk an hour at a moderate to brisk pace, you'll burn 250 to 300 calories. That's about two fried chicken wings or a dozen whole grain crackers or a serving of macaroni and cheese. Low-impact and moderate exercise burns calories, but not a huge amount. Experts say moderate exercise is great for most people's health and for keeping weight off once you've lost it.

More vigorous exercise (like running, aerobic dancing, or high-intensity interval training where your heart rate increases dramatically and you are sweating, breathless, and only able to say a few words at a time) burns many more calories in a shorter period of time and can lead to significant weight loss. Vigorous exercise also provides a great conditioning workout, an emotional high, and more of the many physical and mental benefits of any physical activity. These include lower blood sugar and blood pressure, a boost in HDL (healthy) cholesterol, a stronger cardiovascular system, strengthened muscles, better sleep, and increased circulation. That said, vigorous exercise such as *The Biggest Loser* workouts, Fitness Boot Camps, CrossFit, and other intense programs, are great options if you have a strong fitness base, but they aren't for everyone. Vigorous exercise can cause discomfort and injury, and if you harm yourself, you may not be able to exercise for a long time.

Losing weight from exercise takes exercising intensely for about two hours a day, five days a week. To up your health quotient, any movement is a move in the right direction. So whether you plan to intensify your exercise to become the next "Biggest Loser," or do a little more moderate activity to stay fit or get healthier, both make you the next "Biggest Winner."

Quick-Starts

☐ **Move more.** Any physical activity burns more calories than watching *Magnum* reruns, or for that matter, *The Biggest Loser*. Get up, get out, and move! If you haven't been moving much, start off small like with a daily ten to fifteen minute walk. Then take that walk after as many meals as you can.

☐ **If doing a physical activity where your legs and/or feet are taking a pounding,** like jumping rope or doing jumping jacks, go beyond just wearing supportive shoes. Do it on a supportive floor with some give, not the cement floor in your basement. This will help lessen the chance of developing knee injuries and shin splints.

Your Choice of More How-To's

☐ Manage your expectations for weight loss. Unless your exercise regimen includes vigorous activity, it will help you maintain your weight rather than lose weight.

☐ Decide you're going to make physical activity a priority and schedule it into your week.

☐ To lose weight, look for places in your day where you can cut 300–500 calories. Perhaps replace half the soda you drink with a non-caloric drink or eat half your super-size granola muffin in the morning. Cutting 300–500 calories a day adds up to weight lost each week, each month, each year.

☐ Consider working with a personal trainer who will show you how to exercise properly and keep you motivated. If that's too costly, how about enlisting a buddy to exercise with?

☐ Join a weight loss group like Weight Watchers to feel you're part of a team and have support like *The Biggest Loser* contestants.

For Vigorous Exercisers:

• If just starting out, work with a personal trainer who will teach you how to use equipment properly, how to maintain your form, how many repetitions to do, and keep you safe.

• Work at a variety of intensity levels to tap into different energy systems and work your body in different ways.

• If you're coming back to vigorous activity after taking a break, start out with half your usual workout time for the first week or two and expect an intense level of discomfort during exercise and muscle soreness for days after your workout.

• Join a CrossFit gym or Boot Camp for instruction and to feel you're part of a team.

• If you're looking for inspiration and training to do marathons, long-distance cycling, or triathlons, check out the experts at TeamWILD, teamwild.org.

• Beachbody.com offers many home DVD intense exercise programs. Two that Delaine Wright, exercise physiologist and certified diabetes educator, uses are Insanity and P90X.

• Don't let your ego run your workout. While vigorous exercise is about pushing yourself, trust your gut when enough is enough.

• If you have heart disease or high blood pressure, joint problems or arthritis, or any other injury that may put you at risk, consult your doctor before doing any vigorous activity.

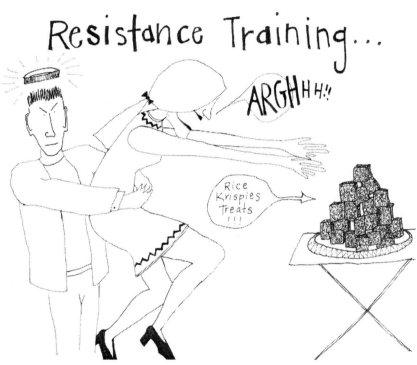

Do #47

Do Some Heavy Breathing and Heavy Lifting

Any type of exercise you do is going to give you health benefits, but we now know that combining aerobic exercise and anaerobic exercise is healthier than doing either one alone. Aerobic exercises are ones that keep you moving, like walking, bicycling, running, swimming, dancing, doing a spin class, hiking, rowing, ice skating, chasing after a frisbee, and household chores like vacuuming and mowing the grass. Anaerobic exercises are short-lasting and of high intensity, like weight machines, resistance bands, calisthenics (push-ups, sit-ups, squats, etc.), free weights, yoga, tai chi, playing tennis or basketball, jumping rope, and rock climbing.

Aerobic exercise helps your circulation, keeps your heart strong, and burns calories. Anaerobic exercise builds or increases your muscle mass, which we tend to lose as we age. It may also help reduce arthritis pain because strong muscles support and protect your joints. Anaerobic exercise can also keep you from becoming frail. Being frail can cause you to fall, especially as you get older. And falls are the leading cause of injury-related death among people sixty-five and older. Plus, if you have pre-diabetes, a recent study conducted with men who did 150 minutes of weight training per week showed a 34 percent lower risk of developing type 2 diabetes.

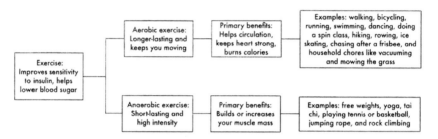

Diagram 2: Difference between aerobic and anaerobic exercise

Anaerobic exercise may also increase the hormones that nourish and protect nerve cells and improve our brain function. In a study with 155 women aged sixty-five to seventy-five at the University of British Columbia at Vancouver, those who participated in a year-long weight training program did 13 percent better when tested for mental function than women who did just stretching and toning exercises.

Together this dynamic duo of aerobic and anaerobic exercise has loads of benefits. They improve your sensitivity to insulin, help lower blood sugar, keep your metabolism burning extra calories after your work out (at rest a pound of muscle burns about six calories while a pound of fat only burns two), strengthen your bones, and keep you physically strong. You may also find you need less medicine when you combine these types of exercise. And of course, like all exercise, they contribute to improving your mood, decrease your risk for certain illnesses, and help with weight loss and/or maintenance.

Quick-Starts

☐ **Get yourself a resistance band and start playing with it.** You can find them online at websites like Amazon or at stores like Target and many others. To get yourself started, watch some resistance band videos. Here are two: video.about.com/exercise/thigh-toning.htm and sparkpeople.com/resource/fitness_articles.asp?id=720.

☐ **See if your health insurance covers a YMCA or gym membership.** If you have a local "Y," they often offer a variety of aerobic and strength training classes, free weights, and resistance training equipment for not a lot of money.

Your Choice of More How-To's

☐ Always warm up before exercising. Muscles work better when they're warm. A ten minute walk will improve blood flow to reduce your risk of injury while working out.

☐ Divide your exercise so you have three to five days of aerobic exercise and two to three days of anaerobic exercise each week. Work up to this in a way that's comfortable for you.

☐ Consider working with a personal trainer, at least for a few sessions, to safely develop a program that's right for your body and your goals. Even just one session can teach you proper form, which may protect you against injury.

☐ Keep yourself safe by getting proper instruction as needed (like when working with resistance machines) and not doing too much too soon.

☐ If you experience muscle soreness, aches, or pains after a workout, this is usually a good thing. Small doses of this type of inflammation leads to greater stamina and strength. To ease the pain, don't apply heat; rather, apply ice, which reduces inflammation.

☐ As you may have read before in other Fitness "How-To's," any activity that causes a sudden increase in blood pressure, like weight lifting, can make retinopathy (a diabetes complication where the blood vessels at the back of your eye become damaged) worse. If you have advanced retinopathy, discuss resistance training activities with your doctor.

Do #48

Respect Your Mother, but Go Ahead and Fidget

Thin people tend to fidget, and fidgeting, would you believe it, burns calories. Scientists have actually studied this and given it a name, Non-Exercise Activity Thermogenesis, or NEAT for short. NEAT consists of low-impact activities like standing, twirling your hair, gesturing (not rudely I hope), tapping your foot, knocking your leg against the table (a colleague of mine always did this and it drove me crazy!), and walking while talking. I suppose chewing gum counts, too.

You may laugh, but these calorie-burners can use up to 350 calories a day. That translates into losing ten to thirty pounds a year. That said, most of us won't lose that kind of weight just from NEAT exercises, but they do add to our overall calorie burn.

Now, get this, new research shows that sitting for long periods of time, like hours behind the computer or TV screen, is harmful. Researchers at the American Cancer Society said sitting down for long periods is as harmful to our bodies as smoking or overexposure to the sun! Extended sitting appears to cause metabolic changes that raise our triglycerides, cholesterol, blood sugar, blood pressure, and appetite. And, we all tend to overestimate how much we actually move throughout the day.

So go ahead and figdet, even to the dismay of your co-workers, and move whether those around you are also moving or not.

Quick-Starts

☐ **Stand while talking on the phone and pace—yes, pace.**

☐ **If you watch TV tonight, hide the remote.** Get up, or at least lean over, to change the channels.

Your Choice of More How-To's

☐ For the girls, do your kegel exercises while in the car waiting for the light to change.

☐ For the guys, squeeze your glutes while in the car staring at the girl waiting at the light.

☐ Wear a wireless telephone headset when you're on the phone and walk around. I do.

☐ Cook while you're watching TV or working at the computer. You'll have to keep getting up to check whatever's on the stove. Just remember to keep a food timer near you, it's saved many a meal for me.

☐ When bringing groceries in from the car, bring in one bag at a time.

☐ Deliver messages to your co-workers in person instead of sending an email.

☐ Laugh more, and more, and more.

☐ Move your hands when you speak—like any good Italian.

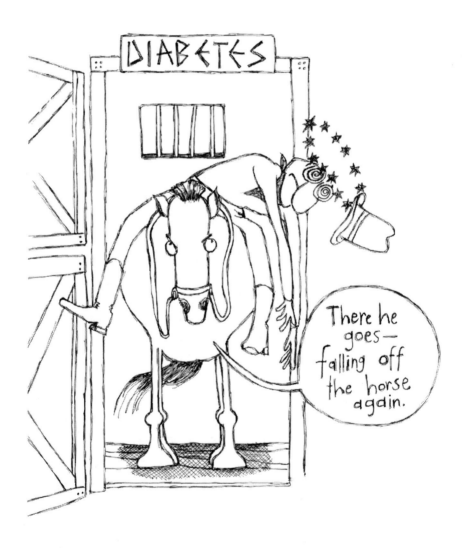

Do #49

Partner with a Friend for Sticking-Power

When I'm giving a talk, I tell people that we are more responsible to others than we are to ourselves—and everyone nods their head. Funny, isn't it? But aren't you more likely to break a promise you make to yourself than one you make to someone else?

One of the best ways to ensure you'll follow through on a regular exercise routine is to have someone exercise with you. Someone who will coax you out of bed and egg you on to work harder or try something new. Someone to huff and puff up the hill with you and celebrate your successes (hopefully with a shopping spree and not an Apple Brown Betty!). Bottom line: research shows buddies who exercise together get better results and have more fun.

Quick-Starts

☐ **Ask someone you know if they'd walk, bicycle, dance, swim, skate, roller blade, play ping pong or scuba dive** with you.

☐ **Join a fitness class or running, walking or bicycling group** where you may meet someone who's also looking for an exercise buddy.

Your Choice of More How-To's

☐ If you belong to a gym, see if they have a sign-up sheet for game partners and fitness pals.

☐ If you're new to a sport, like tennis, sign up for group lessons. You'll meet other people on the same skill level who may want to play with you.

☐ If you're new in town, there are websites where you can find new friends which may lead you to a jogging buddy. Check out ladies-only, GirlfriendSocial.com or co-ed, CompanionTree.com.

☐ Check your neighborhood local paper for running groups.

☐ Search for a "meetup" group online at meetup.com. Local members gather to do a particular physical activity together.

☐ Consider volunteering at your local American Diabetes Association or JDRF office, or a place of worship, where you'll meet new people. One of them may turn out to be your new exercise buddy.

Do #50

De-stress and De-compress

You've probably heard of the "fight" or "flight" response. Your brain thinks you're about to be attacked and your body pumps out stress hormones, like adrenalin and cortisol, to help you run away from the danger. Trouble is, these days much of what we perceive as danger isn't a lion coming at us. Instead, today's stresses come from everyday irritations like getting stuck in traffic, tight deadlines at work, too much to do and too little time to do it, taking care of our family, making ends meet, going through a divorce, or a loved one dying.

When stress hormones are continuously released, our immune system is always in "overdrive," which causes inflammation in the body. Inflammation is unhealthy, and it can lead to heart disease, digestive problems, sleep problems, depression, obesity, and memory problems. And it can raise your blood sugar! Managing your stress is one of the four cornerstones to managing your diabetes—along with healthy eating, being active, and taking your medication.

Quick-Starts

☐ **Take a few slow, deep breaths at various times** throughout the day and get up and stretch.

☐ **Get more sleep.** Sleep does a lot to keep us healthy that we're only now learning about. Most of us need seven to eight hours of sleep a night and few of us get it.

Your Choice of More How-To's

☐ Take a fifteen minute break during the day. Close your door and hang a sign that says, "Gone fishing. Be back at 2 PM." You can read, stare out the window, or just daydream.

☐ Sit or lie comfortably and close your eyes. Place one hand on your belly and notice your breathing. Notice your hand rise and fall with each breath, and feel your body soften into your chair or the floor. Continue until someone knocks on the door or you've taken twenty breaths.

☐ Take a class in a relaxation technique like meditation, yoga, or mindfulness.

☐ Schedule monthly massages, ahhhhhhhh…

☐ Say "No" when there's already too much on your plate.

☐ When you notice anger rising within you, look at your watch or smartphone and wait for ninety seconds to pass. Ninety seconds is the amount of time, according to brain scientist Jill Bolte Taylor, it takes for our stress hormones to surge and pass through and out of our body. At that point, let go of any thoughts of anger, otherwise you will keep stimulating the surge of hormones.

Stress less with these mood enhancers:

• Do any physical activity, including just taking a short walk.

• Do more of what you love, it will keep you healthier—whether it's going to a movie, reading a great book, making Sunday afternoons just about the kids, or finishing the boat you're building in the basement.

• Socialize and connect more with friends.

• Laugh more, it decreases stress hormones.

• Make a play list of your favorite music on your iPod or smartphone. Call it "Stressbuster" and fill it up with the songs that make you sing.

• Stick to your healthy eating. Stress will make you want to reach for the nearest donut, and reaching for the nearest donut may just add to your stress.

• Take the focus off your troubles by volunteering in your community and helping someone else.

• Count your blessings each and every day.

Do #51

Shut Down with Plenty of Shut-Eye

Most of us need seven to eight hours of restful sleep each night to do our best each day. Sleep is the time the body repairs itself. Sleep strengthens our immune system to keep us from getting ill. In fact, if we don't get enough sleep, we are less able to fight off serious illness. People who don't get enough sleep are at a higher risk of dying from heart disease and have higher levels of inflammation and insulin-resistance (the insulin you produce doesn't work well for your body's needs). And people who have type 2 diabetes are already at higher risk for heart attack and stroke, and have insulin-resistance.

Sleep also boosts our brain-power so that we can think more clearly, which is enormously helpful for making good decisions, including those relating to our diabetes care. And sleep keeps our mood up, while lowering our blood pressure, and risk for cancer, heart disease, and weight gain.

Now get this. If you have diabetes, not getting enough sleep can make your sleep even worse. Let me explain. When you don't get enough sleep, it affects hormones that make you hungry the next day, especially for carbohydrates. This leads to a string of unwanted effects: You tend to eat more carbs the day after a sleepless night, which can leave your blood sugar higher before you go to bed. Your kidneys will try to get rid of the extra sugar overnight. How? By waking you up to pee it out!

Well darn, you end up going to the bathroom all night and have another sleepless night!

Researchers say there's also a possible link between diabetes and sleep apnea—a sleep disorder marked by loud snoring followed by gasping or choking sounds as your body stops breathing briefly. The cause of sleep apnea isn't entirely known, but it seems to be connected to two things many people with type 2 diabetes have—insulin-resistance and large amounts of fat around their belly. Sleep apnea can occur hundreds of times during the night, and it's a pretty sure bet that people who suffer from sleep apnea suffer from lousy sleep.

While its importance is often overlooked, a good night's sleep is good medicine for your body, mind, and spirit. You can rest assured of that.

Quick-Starts

☐ **When you go to sleep, keep the bedroom dark and slightly cool,** and keep your feet warm.

☐ **Have a regular sleep pattern every night of the week**. Turn in at the same hour and wake up at the same hour Monday through Sunday.

Your Choice of More How-To's

☐ Drink decaffeinated beverages after mid-afternoon and keep the few hours just before bed free of working out, eating, and drinking alcohol.

☐ Go easy on the alcohol in general, as alcoholic beverages interrupt your sleep and dehydrate you, causing you to wake up groggy. Drinking lots of water before bed helps to dilute the alcohol, but then you'll wake up throughout the night to go to the bathroom!

☐ Relax before going to sleep with a cup of herbal tea, warm milk (with a teaspoon of honey, yum), or a book.

☐ Let your mind wind down before bed by imposing a 9:30 PM curfew on computer and cell phone time and avoiding the 11 o'clock news and late night phone calls from your mother-in-law.

☐ Let technology guide you to sleep. For $2.99, the "Deep Sleep with Andrew Johnson" app may just relax you to sleep. It's available for the iPhone, iPad, Android, and Windows Phone 7. The Sleepsonic Stereo Speaker Pillow, available at sleepsonic.com, is a sound system built into a pillow, and is, as you might expect, more costly.

☐ If you think you may have it, or your wife tells you that you snore like a freight train, get checked for sleep apnea. Untreated sleep apnea is much more dangerous than simply feeling tired the next day. A number of remedies, from weight loss to devices like a CPAP machine or mask, may help open blocked airways while you sleep.

☐ Need I say it? Keep your blood sugars well-controlled.

Do #52

Exercise Your Brain: Be in Learning Mode

Remember who was fighting the War of 1812? Neither do I. A lot of impractical stuff was stuffed into your head in school. Most real learning happens out of school when you get interested in something or have a need to know.

Now it's time to know about diabetes because the more you know, the better you'll do. The fact that you're reading this book already means you want to learn more. And there is always something more to learn. For instance, I recently learned how continuous glucose monitors have become more accurate. That piques my curiosity to try one.

Would you benefit from knowing how to count carbohydrates? Avoid post-meal spikes in your blood sugar? Prevent and manage low blood sugar? Or know which foods you should have always, sometimes, and never? You'll find some of these answers in this book. For others, you will have to look elsewhere, which I encourage you to do.

Also, we're learning we can literally exercise our brains to remain healthier as we age. Doing crossword puzzles and sudoku, and brain fitness programs like the ones from Posit Science, may help improve your memory, eyesight, hearing, and keep you mentally sharp.

The best diabetes students never graduate because they know they can always learn something new that can help them. Plus, exercising your brain keeps it, and you, healthier and more engaged in life.

Quick-Starts

☐ **Check your health insurance policy and see what education it pays for.** Most policies cover a certain amount of hours of education from a reputable organization like the American Diabetes Association (ADA). To see if there's an ADA education program near you, call 1-800-DIABETES (342-2383) or check the ADA website at diabetes.org.

☐ **See if there's a support group in your local community** or a diabetes class you can take at your local hospital, and go.

Your Choice of More How-To's

☐ Ask your health care providers questions during your office visits and, just like in school, write down the answers and re-read them at home.

☐ See if an American Diabetes Association Health Expo is coming to your town. It's a free day of screenings, cooking demonstrations, learning about new products, and leading experts talking about how to care for your diabetes. Check the Expo schedule at diabetes.org/in-my-community/expo/upcoming-expos.html or call 1-800-DIABETES (342-2383).

☐ Attend a Taking Control of Your Diabetes (TCOYD) event if it comes to your town. TCOYD offers one-day learning events across the country. Check their schedule at tcoyd.org.

☐ For intensive, in-residence education, check out the renowned Joslin Diabetes Center. Visit www.joslin.org or call 617-309-2400.

☐ Surf the web for information about diabetes. Here are some trusted websites: the American Diabetes Association at diabetes.org, JDRF at jdrf.org, the Mayo Clinic at mayoclinic.com/health/diabetes/DS01121, WebMD at webmd.com, the National Diabetes Education Program at ndep.nih.gov, and NIDDK at diabetes.niddk.nih.gov.

☐ If you use insulin, or are the parent or caregiver of someone who uses insulin, check out Type 1 University at type1university.com. It's run by my friend, certified diabetes educator Gary Scheiner. You'll find one hour in-depth classes you'll wish someone gave you years ago.

☐ Read diabetes books. They're free in that big building you probably did spend some time in during school, the library. My two other diabetes books, *50 Diabetes Myths That Can Ruin Your Life and the 50 Diabetes Truths That Can Save It* and *The ABCs Of Loving Yourself With Diabetes* may be in your library. If not, they are available on Amazon.com.

☐ Read diabetes magazines. The American Diabetes Association puts out *Forecast*, which is available by subscription and online at forecast. diabetes.org. So are *Diabetes Health* at diabeteshealth.com and *Diabetes Self-Management* at diabetesselfmanagement.com.

☐ Check out Posit Science's brain fitness programs at positscience.com. They show proven benefits for thinking faster, focusing better, remembering more, and sharpening your vision and hearing.

☐ Join a social media or community website like TuDiabetes at tudiabetes.org, Diabetic Connect at diabeticconnect.com, Diabetes Daily at diabetesdaily.com, dLife at dlife.com, A Sweet Life at asweetlife. org, Juvenation at juvenation.org, or pharmaceutical Sanofi's website at diabetes.sanofi.us. These are places to learn and share with others.

☐ Check out patient blogs online by googling "diabetes blogs," and my own informational articles on *The Huffington Post* at huffingtonpost .com/riva-greenberg/#blogger_bio.

☐ Mentor someone else with diabetes. You learn when you teach.

Shared Learning

Since we learn from each other, here are some personal "How-To's" from people living with diabetes:

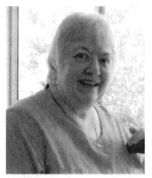

Lynda

I have a book-rack on my stationary bike in my bedroom so I can accomplish two things at the same time. First thing in the morning when I get up, I do my daily devotions, or read a book, and exercise.

— **Lynda Sardeson**
65 years old, living with diabetes 20 years.

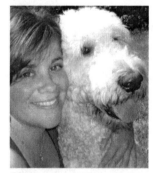

Ginger

I go outside into the woods with my dogs every morning. I made a rule for myself that I will not go until I have first checked my blood sugar. So, I get my exercise and ensure I have done my morning check.

— **Ginger Vieira**
27 years old, living with diabetes 13 years.

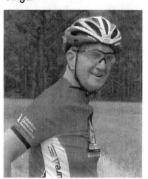

Tom

I mark when I do an activity on my calendar. I use "Ky" for kayak, "B" for bike, "Kt" for stunt kite flying, "Gf" for golf, "Gd" for Golds Gym, "Y" for yard work, "H" for hike, and leave a blank if I take a day off, which is necessary! This way I have a quick glance at the end of the month of my activity.

— **Tom Fineco**
73 years old, living with diabetes 20 years.

Your Quick-Start "Do" Sheet

Use this worksheet to help you accomplish any Fitness "Do" in a way that works best for you.

The "Do" I will do is:

_____

_____

_____

Why it's important to me to do this:

_____

_____

_____

My "How-To" is/are:

_____

_____

_____

When I will begin:

_____

_____

_____

How often I will do this:

_____

_____

_____

Where I will do this:

_____

_____

_____

Who can support me:

_____

_____

_____

What can stop me:

_____

_____

_____

What I will do about that:

_____

_____

_____

What was successful and how I can keep doing it:

_____

_____

_____

Attitude Do's

If you do your best, or close to it, most of the time,
you'll be happy, or close to it, more of the time.

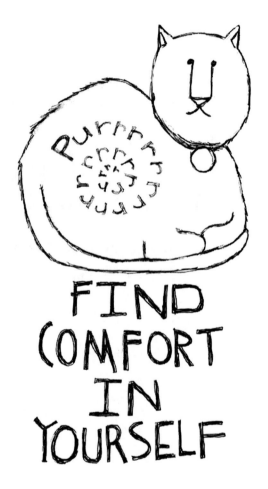

FIND
COMFORT
IN
YOURSELF

Do #53

Know You're the Most Important Member of Your Medical Team

Here's the sometimes harsh, yet also powerful, truth: we are each the captain of our diabetes ship. While you may spend a dozen hours a year with your health care providers (and that would be on the high side), that leaves 8,724 hours you spend on your own managing your diabetes. As you become more responsible for your diabetes and take good care of yourself, chances are you will become healthier and diabetes will feel less of a burden.

Bottom line, it's not up to your health care providers to keep you healthy, with your help. It's up to you to keep yourself healthy, with their help.

Quick-Starts

☐ **Ask your doctor for a referral to a certified diabetes educator (CDE).** This is a professional who is specifically trained in helping you manage your diabetes. You can also find a CDE near you on the American Association of Diabetes Educators website at www.diabeteseducator.org/DiabetesEducation/Find.html. A diabetes educator can teach you everything you need to know about managing your diabetes.

☐ **Think about why it's important to you to be healthy.** Maybe it's to spend more time with your grandchildren or doing a hobby you love. When you reflect on your "meaningful reason" to be healthy, you'll be more inspired to take care of yourself.

Your Choice of More How-To's

☐ If you've been wishing, hoping, praying, or begging for your diabetes to go away, accept that it's not going to happen. It's time to take the wheel of your ship—and your power—back by doing those things necessary to take care of your diabetes.

☐ Be an active partner with your doctors. Write down your blood sugars at home when you check and bring the results to your office visit. When you get lab tests, ask what the results mean and what you should do about them.

☐ Check out PatientsLikeMe.com, a health information sharing website. Patients post their personal stories and medical information to share ideas, experiences, and learning with other patients like themselves. It's a valuable resource for caregivers and medical practitioners, too.

☐ Learn more about diabetes. See "Do #52. Exercise Your Brain: Be In Learning Mode" for many recommended resources including informational websites, community sites, books, and magazines.

☐ If you have type 1 diabetes, check out this social networking and resource website that has an exceptionally positive attitude, Welcometotype1.com.

Do #54

Be a Warrior, Not a Worrier

Every day we walk a line between being a warrior and a worrier in how we manage our diabetes. It's so easy to be a worrier. After all, there seems to be an awful lot to worry about: Will I get complications? Will they get worse? Why did my doctor just add another pill to my treatment plan? It's easy to worry when we're afraid, don't have enough information, or get frustrated by all the work diabetes takes.

We become warriors when we have good information to manage our diabetes and know that it's up to us to take responsibility for ourselves and our health. And know that the benefit can be a longer, healthier life. See your diabetes as a wake-up call to get healthier. If you weren't that healthy before you got diabetes, here's an opportunity to make a fresh start. Millions of people have made it their fresh start.

You might also see your diabetes as life's way of asking, "Am I satisfied with my life or is there something more I want to do or be?" Many people have found a greater sense of meaning and purpose in their lives because of getting diabetes. At every moment, in this very moment, you can choose to be a warrior or worrier.

Quick-Starts

☐ **This week commit to one small step you will take to manage your diabetes a little better.** Choose a "Do" and "How-To" from this book that you like! Perhaps your small step will be to check your blood sugar two more times this week or schedule a doctor visit you know is overdue.

☐ **Every day notice something you did to take care of your diabetes,** and just take a moment to appreciate your effort.

Your Choice of More How-To's

☐ Focus on what you want, not on what you don't want. For example, see in your mind's eye your ideal you—how you'd like to look and feel. Then take one small action to move you closer to your picture.

☐ Keep your focus off the things you don't want to have happen, like complications. It will only steal your energy and call out your Worrier. When you find yourself thinking about worrisome things, search your mind for something that you are doing well with your diabetes.

☐ Connecting with your Warrior is about following your heart and not your fear. There are two keys to following your heart—having the discipline to listen to the voice inside you and the courage to follow it.

☐ Schedule activities that make you happy. When you're happier, you have more strength and energy to manage your diabetes.

☐ Think about times when you've overcome a challenge before. What did you do? How did you do it? What strengths did you use—maybe courage, persistence, asking for help, learning something new? How can you use your strengths now to help you manage your diabetes a little better?

Do #55

Aim for Better, Not Perfect

Here's why: trying to be perfect managing your diabetes will drive you insane! Nobody manages diabetes perfectly. You can't always know what your body's doing and you can't always control it. Even if you do the same exact things two days in a row, you won't get the same exact results. The good news is that you don't have to be perfect. Studies show that when it comes to delaying or preventing diabetes complications, the benefit of having an A1C (average blood sugar measurement over the past two to three months) closer to the high end of normal, 6%, as opposed to 6.5%, is very small. So, forget perfect. Just try to make small improvements.

Now that you know you don't have to be perfect, did you know that it's good to take "diabetes vacations" now and then? Psychologist and certified diabetes educator Bill Polonsky says we should. They help us to not get burned out. Diabetes vacations are pretty much what you would imagine, a very short break, like skipping a diabetes task you do regularly once in a while. For instance, you might take every Friday night off from your diabetes-friendly meal plan. Taking diabetes vacations actually helps you let go of stress, restore your energy, and manage your diabetes for the years to come. Just make sure your diabetes vacation is short and safe. A diabetes vacation should never put you at risk.

Quick-Starts

☐ **One day of the week, treat yourself to a meal that's not on your meal plan.**

☐ **Ask a loved one to do something for you this week** like shopping for groceries or bringing you your meter and strips when you're lounging in bed. That's my idea of a glorious diabetes vacation.

Your Choice of More How-To's

☐ Forget perfection. Instead see the things you're doing well.

☐ Work with your health care provider to make sure your "diabetes vacations" are safe and that you and your diabetes don't suffer.

☐ Pick one day of the week to not do a diabetes task that doesn't put you at risk, like skipping your walk when you really don't feel like it.

☐ If you're a parent of a child with diabetes, you also need to to take occasional breaks, says certified diabetes educator Betty Brackenridge. Develop a support circle of extended family members and good friends who can pitch in, perhaps with blood sugar checks or cooking a meal.

☐ Diabetes vacations should be short. If you find you're not doing what you should to take care of your diabetes, seek professional help to get you back on track and on your treatment plan.

what goes on in a diabetic's head:

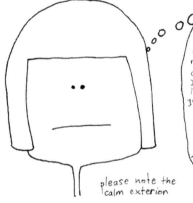

please note the calm exterion

Do #56

~~Test~~ Check Your Blood Sugar, but Don't Keep Score

Diabetes can seem like a life of numbers: blood sugar numbers, blood pressure numbers, cholesterol numbers. Then we often judge those numbers, and ourselves, as "good" and "bad." But these judgments won't help us do better, and most of the time they will make us feel worse. In the past, my heart would race with frustration, disappointment, and a sense that I had failed when a number like 250 mg/dl (13.8 mmol/l) appeared on my glucose meter. Forget it! Today I see (mostly) the number and think what may have caused it. See your numbers as they are meant to be seen—information, not a judgment of your self-worth.

You may notice in the headline of this "Do" that this is the only place in the book where I say "test" your blood sugar. You will often see the word "test" used for checking your blood sugar. But "testing" sounds like we're being graded, which means we either pass or fail. What we're really doing is "checking" our blood sugar so we know where we are and how things like food, exercise, stress, and our medicine influence the numbers we get.

When you check your blood sugar and it's out of your target range, think what may have caused it. Think what you can do a little differently next time to get in, or closer to, your target range. When we look at our numbers that way, we can make the adjustments that will help us stay in our target range more often.

Quick-Starts

☐ **Keep your expectations realistic and don't beat yourself up.** No matter what you do, you won't always get the numbers you expect. That's diabetes.

☐ **Give yourself the same care and compassion you would a good friend** when you're struggling with your diabetes. When you treat yourself kindly, you're better able to tap into your strength and abilities to manage your diabetes.

Your Choice of More How-To's

☐ Reward your effort not your outcome. You can't always control what the result of your action will be, but you can control making the effort.

☐ Whatever number comes up on your meter, think why you might have gotten that number. For instance, if the number is lower than your target range, ask yourself, "Did I skip a meal or snack? Did I exercise more than I thought I would? Did I incorrectly guess the amount of carbohydrates in my meal or the carbohydrate exchanges?" And, if the number is higher than your target range, ask yourself, "Did I under-count the carbs in that scrumptious peanut butter chocolate chip caramel cookie? Did I skip my run because Aunt Mary showed up unannounced this morning!?" Whatever the answer, use this information to do a little better next time.

Do #57

Cancel Diabetes Fright-Nights

I won't deny it, diabetes can be scary at times. High blood sugar, over time, can damage much of your body. You may feel tingling or burning in your feet, or feel no sensation at all. You may have vision problems or lose your vision. You may get infections that don't heal, find your kidneys weaken, have sexual problems, or be more prone to heart disease. Nerve damage can even make food move more slowly through your stomach, which throws off the timing of your medication. All of these ailments are called diabetes complications (see "Do #22. Know How To Delay or Prevent Diabetes Complications").

But here's the fine print, what you hardly ever hear or read about but need to know. Diabetes complications largely occur when your blood sugar is not well-controlled. In other words, they come from *poorly managed* diabetes. Well-managed diabetes can prevent, delay, and possibly reverse diabetic complications. Well-managed diabetes, as leading diabetes educator and psychologist Bill Polonsky says, is the leading cause of nothing. I like to say it can be a leading cause of happiness.

Even though I've had diabetes for forty years, I am convinced I would not be as healthy as I am today if I had never gotten it. It motivates me to keep my weight in check, take my walk every day, and visit my doctors regularly. Diabetes has also become my work. It gives me enormous pleasure to help others with diabetes, and it gives me my sense of purpose in the world.

Can you use your diabetes to motivate you to get healthier, and appreciate how many wonderful things you have?

Quick-Starts

☐ **Do mini-relaxation activities when you're frightened.** You can sit quietly, close your eyes, and repeat the sound "ohm" in your head for two minutes. Or take five to ten deep, slow breaths for instant relaxation.

☐ **If you're worried about something specific, get it checked right away.** For instance, if you notice a new feeling, or lack of feeling, in your feet, make an appointment today to see your doctor or podiatrist (foot doctor).

Your Choice of More How-To's

☐ If you feel a general sense of anxiety, or feel frightened of what may lie ahead, getting more information about what concerns you can lower your distress.

☐ If you experience a setback, take a small step to improve your diabetes care. Action helps us feel less scared and helpless.

☐ Make sure you have a realistic treatment plan with steps that you can follow. If not, work with your provider to create one.

☐ When a fright night is upon you, lift your mood by shifting your energy. Take a walk, go to a movie, or play some favorite music.

☐ You can play a game and learn to quiet your fears. "DiabetesIQ" is a free app that works on an iPhone, iPad, iPod Touch, and with Android compatible smartphones and tablets. This app tests your diabetes knowledge through fun quizzes and visual puzzles and lets you compare your results with others' in real time.

Do #58

Know that Your Diabetes is Only About You

Nobody has your hips, your eyes, your lips, or your diabetes. Like a masterwork, you are unique and so is your diabetes. I once went on a long weekend with two female friends who also have type 1 diabetes. We each ate exactly the same meals and did the same exercise, and we each got different numbers checking our blood sugar throughout the day. There's no value in comparing yourself to others, honestly. It bummed you out in high school and it will only confuse you now.

There is one way, however, in which your diabetes isn't just about you: it affects those who love you. Bear in mind that they have your best interest at heart even when they're yelling at you not to eat that piece of chocolate cake, or asking you every time you turn around, "What's your blood sugar?" Be open with your loved ones, share your feelings, and let them also express their feelings. While your diabetes is only about you, it affects them too.

Quick-Starts

☐ **Know that your treatment plan, your medicines, and your lab reports** are all unique to you because diabetes works differently in each of us.

☐ **If you don't know how the foods you eat affect your blood sugar, keep a record this week.** Write down your meals, check your blood sugar before and two hours after you take your first bite of food, and write down your numbers. If you need help figuring out what your numbers mean, bring your record to your doctor and have him explain how food impacts your blood sugar.

Your Choice of More How-To's

☐ Check your blood sugar before and after you exercise and write down your numbers. You'll see the impact of exercise on your blood sugar.

☐ Get to know how stress affects your blood sugar by checking it when you feel stressed. Most people find stress makes their blood sugar go up, but some people find it goes down. Every time I give a presentation, my blood sugar goes up!

☐ Let your loved ones know that you appreciate their love and support, and find a quiet fifteen minutes to discuss with them how they can best help you if they're not doing it now, and how you can make it easier for them. Diabetes affects all of you.

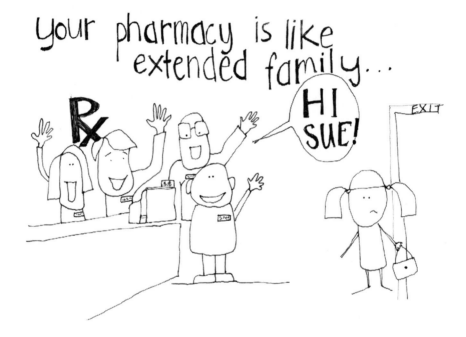

Do #59

Develop a Personal Support Network

All of us manage our diabetes better with support. If you have one or more people in your circle who can help you, you'll find diabetes much easier to live with. Maybe a family member or friend can lend a hand shopping for, or cooking, healthy meals. Maybe they will go for a walk with you or drive you to a doctor's appointment. Or carry glucose tablets in their pockets like my husband does for me. Or just lend an ear when you feel overwhelmed. Yes, he does that, too. Studies show that having friends, support, and strong social ties can improve your blood pressure, memory, overall health, and longevity. At the same time, it can decrease physical ailments, mental decline, depression, and Alzheimer's.

I have one more point to make here: your personal support network should also include you. It's so easy to beat ourselves up when we make a mistake with our diabetes or fall short of our goals. Like when we don't get ourselves out the door for that walk, we get a blood sugar number that we don't like, or we eat that donut we told ourselves we wouldn't.

If you treat yourself with compassion, you'll actually do better than if you guilt-trip yourself for messing up. Jean Fain, a psychotherapist and teaching associate at Harvard Medical School, says "self-compassion is the missing ingredient in every diet and weight-loss plan." In a study with eighty-four women, those who were dieting and were taught self-compassion ate less than the women who felt guilty about eating "forbidden foods." No matter what, we each deserve to be our own best friend.

Quick-Starts

☐ **Use this easy, free app from EatSmart™ to learn, in minutes, how to develop your own personal support network.** I created these and you'll find them at eatsmart.quantiacare.com under "Build Your Personal Support Network." They're also available as a free app for iPhone, iPod touch, iPad, and Android.

☐ **Join one of the many online diabetes communities** like tudiabetes. org, diabeticconnect.com, diabetessisters.org (just for females), juvenation. org, or myglu.org. (The last two are specifically for people with type 1 diabetes.) These are great places to chat with others and find support.

Your Choice of More How-To's

☐ Your health care team is a part of your support network. If you need a little more help with your diabetes management, ask your health care provider for a referral to a diabetes educator. This is a medical professional who specializes in diabetes care. (You can also locate a diabetes educator in your area at www.diabeteseducator.org/DiabetesEducation/Find.html.) If you need help with meal planning or carbohydrate counting, ask your health care provider for a referral to a dietitian.

☐ Think of a small, specific way a family member or friend can help you and then ask for that help.

☐ Do something where you'll meet new people—take a class, volunteer at your church. You may make a new friend or acquaintance there.

☐ Go to a diabetes support group meeting. Your local American Diabetes Association or JDRF office can help you find one.

Do #60

Make "I'm Grateful" a Daily Mantra

Studies show that if you pause to consciously experience and express gratefulness, you will tend to heal faster, manage problems more easily, have a stronger immune system, and find life more satisfying. Trust me, as Oprah Winfrey says, this is what I know for sure: when you spend more time being appreciative, non-judging, loving, playful, patient, forgiving, and grateful, you will be healthier and happier and find diabetes easier to manage and live with.

Quick-Starts

☐ **Do an act of kindness.** It can be planned, like helping out a friend or neighbor when they ask, or random, like letting someone go in front of you at the check-out line because they're in a rush. Being kind to others creates good feelings for both you and the person you are kind to.

☐ **Each evening before you go to sleep and/or each morning before you greet the day, think of three things you're grateful for** or that went well in the last twenty-four hours. They can be large or small. For instance, the simple joy of seeing a child playing, a secret smile you shared with your partner, a blessedly quiet evening alone at home with a great book, or backing your new Porsche off the dealer's lot.

Your Choice of More How-To's

☐ Keep a Gratitude Journal and write three to five things a week that you're thankful for. Keep it short and keep your entries new. People who do this report feeling happier with fewer physical problems. Grateful people also report they do more physical activity, sleep longer, and feel more refreshed.

☐ Write a letter to someone who had a positive impact on your life. Then either mail the letter or even better, deliver it and read it in person.

☐ Do something for others who are less fortunate. It's an easy way to feel grateful for what you have.

Shared Learning

Since we learn from each other, here are some personal "How-To's" from people living with diabetes:

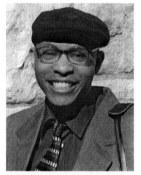

Reggie

I've always been an optimistic person, but on those "not so good days" I get my motivation from others and my family. I volunteer, mentor, and try to inspire others. If I can make someone smile or they give me a hug, I feel good. My positive attitude is a part of managing my diabetes along with doing things I just want to try, which I've put on my "bucket list."

— **Reggie Bishop**
47 years old, living with diabetes 39 years.

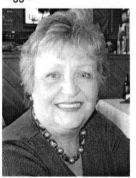

Denise

Sometimes I just have to push myself off the pity pot. When I am doing all the right things and getting the wrong results, I reach out to my friends and the community. I hosted ten women at a fundraising luncheon for a women's shelter and it made me so happy! Diabetes is not just about following a diet or dealing with my weight, but a way of caring for myself.

— **Denise Costabile**
58 years old, living with diabetes two years.

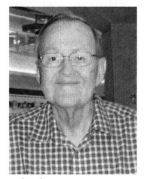

Richard

I communicate with many friends online in diabetes support groups and on Facebook. It is very rewarding to help and inspire other people with diabetes, especially the parents of diabetic children.

— **Richard Vaughn**
72 years old, living with diabetes 66 years.

Your Quick-Start "Do" Sheet

Use this worksheet to help you accomplish any Attitude "Do" in a way that works best for you.

The "Do" I will do is:

_____

_____

_____

Why it's important to me to do this:

_____

_____

_____

My "How-To" is/are:

_____

_____

_____

When I will begin:

_____

_____

_____

How often I will do this:

_____

_____

_____

Where I will do this:

_____

_____

_____

Who can support me:

_____

_____

_____

What can stop me:

_____

_____

_____

What I will do about that:

_____

_____

_____

What was successful and how I can keep doing it:

_____

_____

_____

TRU FOR WE.

(Hold under chin while looking in mirror)

Bonus Do's

Here are five more "Do's"
that will make you extra successful!

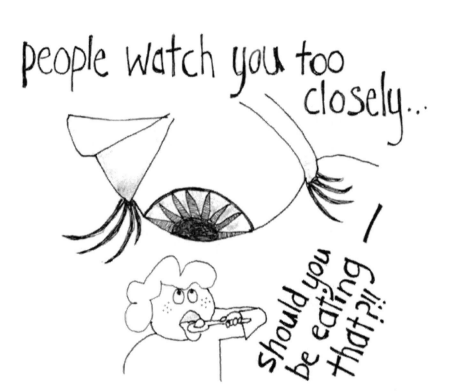

1. Make a Citizen's Arrest if You Have "Diabetes Police" in Your Life

"Diabetes Police" are, according to psychologist and diabetes educator Bill Polonsky, usually our family members and friends. They might be your husband, wife, child, Aunt Matilda, neighbor, or the gal you always run into in the office kitchen. Out of fear or worry, they nag you or find fault with how you take care of your diabetes. For instance, just as you begin to put something really yummy into your mouth, they gasp, wag their finger, and say, "You can't eat that!" Actually, you probably can, just not as much or as often as you'd like. Try to remember your loved ones love you and their nagging is their way of showing their concern.

When I first got married, after taking care of my diabetes by myself for thirty years, my husband would follow me into the kitchen to see what number would come up on my glucose meter when I did my morning check. What if a "bad" number came up? (I was not quite as enlightened as I am today about numbers not being "good" or "bad.")

I shooed him away a few times until I realized it wasn't a good way to start a marriage. So I let him stand there, which he did about five times, and I used that time to talk with him about diabetes, how it works and why I thought I got the number I got. When he had satisfied his curiosity about the meter, he asked me what he could do that would help me. I told him, "Tell me when you read something new related to diabetes" and "Just listen to me when I'm having an awful diabetes-day." He does, and it makes me feel supported, and him feel valued.

Quick-Starts

☐ **Let your diabetes police know that you appreciate their concern** but what they're doing isn't helpful. Instead, tell them what they can do that will help you.

☐ **If your diabetes police are right about what you're doing—or not doing**—thank them for their concern and consider how you might improve what you're doing.

Your Choice of More How-To's

☐ If your diabetes police don't realize most of the time you handle your diabetes well, set them straight—in the nicest way, of course.

☐ Thanks to the Behavioral Diabetes Institute, you can give your loved ones a little fold-out Diabetes Etiquette Card that will help them know just how they can help you and what is just downright annoying! You can download it at http://www.behavioraldiabetesinstitute .org/resources-diabetes-information-publications-etiquettecard.html, or call 858-336-8693. If you are a health care professional, you can contact your local Accu-Chek representative for free copies.

☐ If *you* are the "Diabetes Police," ask your loved one how you can help them. Also, let them know that you care about them and understand that living with diabetes is a lot to deal with.

2. Set Yourself, and Your Home, Up for Success

There's a saying I often hear: "People will make the healthy choice when the healthy choice is the easy choice." It's true, and there are things you can do to make healthy choices easier. Set up your home, and your day, in ways that help you to eat healthy, move more, take your medicine, check your blood sugar, and lessen the stress in your life. Willpower is not what's going to get you to the finish line with diabetes, because willpower runs out. Making it easier to make healthy choices is how to set yourself up for success.

All the "How-To's" in this book are steps to success. Here are a few more that either bear repeating or haven't been said before.

Quick-Starts

☐ **Go shopping with a list of healthy groceries to buy and stick to your list.** Also, go shopping when you're not hungry. Otherwise, you'll find you're tempted to throw unhealthy foods into your cart.

☐ **Put your food into a bowl.** Don't stand at the fridge eating one spoonful after another from the ice cream container, or eat handful after handful out of the cereal box or pretzel bag. Instead, put a serving size into a bowl. When you've come to the bottom, you're done.

Your Choice of More How-To's

☐ Write out one or two goals you want to achieve to do a little better with your diabetes care. Then write down a few action steps for each. Make your actions very specific: what you will do, how much, how long, when, and why. Or use the worksheet at the back of this book to start working on a goal.

☐ Share your goal and action steps from above with someone you trust who will support your efforts. I call that person a "blood sugar buddy." Once a week spend fifteen minutes and share the progress you've made toward your goal. Having someone check on our progress usually keeps us more motivated.

☐ Keep a journal and write in it when you're stressed. Often writing about our feelings helps us feel more calm. And, when you're less stressed, you have more energy and focus to make smart and healthy decisions about your diabetes.

☐ Listen to your body before you eat something. Ask yourself, "Am I really hungry or frustrated or restless? Am I hungry or actually thirsty?" Often our body is just asking for water. Above all, listen to your body before you take action.

☐ Take rests when you're tired and do fun stuff in between working hard at your diabetes. You deserve to enjoy yourself and it'll help you keep going.

Ways to make yourself successful:

• Make small changes, one small change at a time. For instance, add one serving of fruits or vegetables to any of your meals this week. When you make changes one at a time and make them small, you'll have a bigger chance for success.

• Do one thing at a time and give it your full attention. Living as we do with constant multi-tasking, we do many things without thinking that often don't support our health. Focus fully on whatever you're doing at the moment. You'll be more aware of your actions, more productive, and more successful at whatever you do.

• Eat, exercise, and sleep about the same amount and about the same time of day, every day. Your body loves regularity and will be more healthy for it.

• Ask for help. For instance, have a friend come over and help you clear your kitchen of junk food or go to the supermarket together and read nutrition labels.

• Stay positive by looking at what you've accomplished, no matter what it is. Know that wherever you are is okay and that you will continue to take steps forward.

Setting up your home for success:

• Keep your fridge and your pantry stocked with fresh foods, not junk food. That way, when you're hungry, you'll have healthy foods at the ready.

• Keep a bowl of fresh fruit on your kitchen counter. You'll be more likely to grab one of these rather than demolish a bag of potato chips from the pantry.

• If you have exercise equipment in your home: 1) remove clothes hanging on equipment; 2) place equipment in front of a TV; 3) find a ten to fifteen minute window in your day to use the equipment—and use it!

• Use visual cues to help you:

  ○ Lay out exercise clothes before you go to bed so when you wake up you'll be reminded to work out.

○ Keep your medicines where you can see them.

○ Keep your calendar with doctor appointments written in it close at hand.

○ Keep a log book beside your meter to record your blood sugar results.

• Post reminders for things you want to start or continue, otherwise they're easy to forget.

• Cut pictures out of a magazine of who you'd like to be. Pictures that reflect the body, energy, and spirit you'd like to have, how you'd like to be living, and what you'd love to be doing. Paste them into a collage and hang it where you'll see it. Look at it often. Subconsciously, you'll begin to do the behaviors that will lead you to your ideal you.

3. Develop Healthy Habits to Save Time and Effort

If you develop some healthy habits to take care of your diabetes, you'll find it easier and quicker to do your diabetes tasks. Habits are short-cuts. They help us do things with less thought, time, and effort. For instance, you're more likely to exercise regularly if you exercise at the same time each day or have a standing date with an exercise buddy. You may eat less at meals if you get in the habit of using smaller plates. One of my healthy habits is checking my blood sugar first thing when I wake up in the morning and every night just before I go to bed. I don't give it a thought, I just do it. I also keep my glucose meter in the same place all the time, on my kitchen counter. This way I never have to look for it, which saves me time and headaches. A woman I interviewed told me she keeps her meter in a bright pink case in her purse so it's easy to find. That helps her check more often.

Psychologists tell us that we form new habits by doing something over and over for about a month. While most of us have developed some unhealthy habits over the years, it's never too late to develop healthier habits.

Quick-Starts

☐ **Think about what small things you can do in your day to make your diabetes care easier.** For instance, would it help you to keep glucose tablets on your bedside table? Can you set up a way to remind yourself to always check your blood sugar before you exercise or drive? Can you create the habit of always eating breakfast?

☐ **Tell someone about the habit you want to develop.** Sometimes just telling another person, or saying it out loud, gives you more motivation.

Your Choice of More How-To's

☐ Several times a day hold a picture in your mind of you performing a new habit. See it like a small movie. See every step you're doing. Make it as clear as you can.

☐ Replace an unhealthy habit. For instance, if you find yourself lighting up a cigarette, stop and do something different. Take a walk instead.

☐ Find a trigger for a new behavior. For instance, I keep my long-acting insulin pen in a cup and every morning take it out of the cup to signal me to take my injection.

☐ Ask your health care provider or diabetes educator to work with you to come up with healthy habits that can support your diabetes care.

☐ Keep reminders around for a month to practice your habit: put up sticky notes, schedule a reminder on your computer, set an alarm on your smartphone.

☐ Feedback often helps people perform and stick with a new habit. For instance:

○ If you want to start an exercise habit, a simple pedometer that measures your steps may encourage you. Or if you're looking for something with more bells and whistles, try Striiv. Available at www. striiv.com, Striiv makes a game out of walking, running, and climbing stairs. You'll get points and trophies for what you accomplish.

○ Weighing yourself once a week may help you stick to your healthy meal plan. After years of not weighing myself, now I do it every Tuesday morning before breakfast. When I see my weight's up a little, I get back on track quickly.

○ Using a blood pressure monitor regularly at home can remind you to cut down on salt in your diet.

4. Know How To Get Medicines and Supplies Covered if Money is Tight

If you don't have health insurance, you may be able to get some of your medicines, supplies, and education classes paid for by programs offered by the government and many pharmaceutical companies. Medicare is also available to people who are sixty-five years of age and older or people who are under sixty-five but have certain disabilities.

Quick-Starts

☐ **Get prescriptions filled at local chain stores.** Many, such as Walmart, Walgreens, Target, and Duane Reade, offer prescription assistance programs and discount cards that make drugs available at lower prices.

☐ **If you're on a Medicare drug plan, use the mail-order pharmacy.** It's cheaper than buying your medicines at a drug store or chain store's pharmacy.

Your Choice of More How-To's

☐ Call Medicare at 800–633–4227 and see what it offers. Typically, Medicare covers the cost of glaucoma screening and check-ups with a podiatrist (foot doctor), including special shoes, orthotics, and corrective shoe inserts.

☐ If you don't have health care insurance, or need financial help to pay for your diabetes care, you can find information at: diabetes.niddk.nih. gov/dm/pubs/financialhelp.

☐ Check the Partnership for Prescription Assistance at pparx.org or call 1-888-477-2669 to see if you're eligible for free or discounted medicines.

☐ Get the Together Rx Access Card that offers 25 to 40 percent off brand-name prescription medications at pharmacies nationwide. Call 1-800-444-4106 or go to togetherrxaccess.com.

☐ Check out these discount programs online: Lilly Cares offers discounts on Humalog insulin, Novo Nordisk's Cornerstones4Care offers discounts on Levemir and Novolog insulin, and Sanofi's Patient Connection program offers free or low-cost Lantus and Apidra insulins. Freestyle offers its Promise program, which gives a discount on test strips.

☐ Call your city, county, or state health department to see if there are local programs to help with health care or medications.

☐ You can visit the US government's health care website, healthcare. gov, to find out about insurance options and laws that may affect your coverage.

Ask your health care provider if she can:

- Prescribe a generic, rather than a brand name, medicine. Generics cost less.
- Work with you on a sliding scale for the cost of office visits.
- Provide free samples of medicines or supplies.
- Tell you when is the best time to check your blood sugar so you can use fewer test strips yet get the information you need to manage your blood sugar.

• Guide you to any free or low-cost clinics in your community or pharmaceutical programs that provide medicines and/or supplies for free or at lower costs. For example, Roche Diagnostics' patient assistance program offers free glucometers and medications to individuals who are unable to pay and are not eligible for public or private coverage.

Call the American Diabetes Association's national call center at 1-800-DIABETES (342-2383) or check the ADA website at diabetes.org to find out:

• About affordable health insurance.

• How to save money on medicines and supplies.

• Where to get financial assistance for complications such as kidney disease and prosthetics for amputees.

• Where to find supplies and free or low-cost health insurance for children under age 18.

5. Travel Smart and Travel Safe

I travel often both for business and pleasure, and there are many "rules of the road" that will help you travel safely with diabetes and make sure all your diabetes gear ends up with you when you arrive. First, I start out with a packing list. It has all my medications and supplies on it, and I refer to it before every trip.

Below are some guidelines for safe and smart travel, including what you can bring and how to get through airport security relatively smoothly and leave those security workers smiling.

Quick-Starts

☐ **Always take your diabetes supplies and medicines on board the airplane with you.** You don't want to discover they're in the bag the airline lost. Also, the cargo hold may damage them due to changes in temperature.

☐ **Carry a doctor's note with you that says you have diabetes.** If you use insulin and needles to treat your diabetes, carry a note explaining that, too.

Your Choice of More How-To's

☐ Pack twice the amount of medicine and supplies you'll need and separate them in two bags. That way if one of your bags gets lost or stolen, you'll still have what you need.

☐ Make sure you have enough medicine to last while you'll be away. If not, get extra before you go.

☐ If you take insulin, talk to your health care provider about how to time your injections if you are going to cross time zones. To be honest, I've never quite figured this out. I test my blood sugar every few hours the first two to three days I'm in a new time zone and adjust my insulin dose and frequency to stay in or near my target range.

☐ Never let your insulin get too hot or too cold. Keep it out of the sun and out of the glove compartment and trunk of your car. If you're going to Tucson, Arizona in August, as I did, put it in a Frio bag. Frio bags keep insulin at a safe, cool temperature without the need for ice packs or refrigeration. They're available at www.frioinsulincoolingcase.com.

☐ Always bring food or a snack with you. You can never tell when you'll need food and it won't be available—other than giant Cinnabons. Truly, the smell of those cinnamon buns at almost every airport would tempt even the most devoted health fanatic.

☐ Wear some form of diabetes medical identification and/or carry a card in your wallet (see "Do #40. Add a Medical Alert Bracelet to Your Jewelry Collection").

☐ If you wear an insulin pump, carry the phone number for the manufacturer. If something happens to your pump, many insulin pump companies will offer a loaner pump or get you what you need right away. Also have short- and long-acting insulins with you in case your pump malfunctions.

When flying:

• You can call the TSA's helpline, "TSA Cares," established to assist passengers with medical conditions and disabilities prior to getting to the airport. The toll free number is: 1-855-787-2227. You'll also find information at tsa.gov/travelers/airtravel/disabilityandmedicalneeds.

• You can bring necessary liquids like glucose gels, juice, and fruit drinks in quantities larger than three ounces. Just let the security workers know that it's for your diabetes.

• If you're carrying syringes, insulin pens, or lancets (used for checking blood sugar), they must have a cap on them.

• If you use insulin, you need to carry a pharmaceutical label for it. In my wallet I carry the side of the insulin box that shows the insulin's name and my name.

• If you're carrying a glucagon emergency kit, it should be in its original container with the pharmaceutical label.

• Carry a prescription for your medications just in case you lose them—or your glass insulin vial falls off the table, lands on the floor, and splits into a thousand pieces, with its precious liquid seeping into the floorboards as you stare in shock and dismay.

• You are allowed to bring insulin and insulin-dispensing devices (like insulin pens and syringes), lancets, glucose meters, test strips, an insulin pump and pump supplies, a glucagon emergency kit, and urine ketone test strips. You're also allowed to transport used syringes in a sharps disposal container.

• Airport X-ray machines won't hurt your glucose meter, insulin, or insulin pump. However, here are some tips to be extra careful with your insulin pump:

  ○ If wearing your pump through the metal detector, hold it over your belly button. That gives you the greatest chance of not setting off the alarm. Who knew?

- Request a pat down instead of going through the whole body screen machine with your pump. If you don't want to go through the metal detector, you can also request a body pat-down.

- If you're being wanded, hold your pump away from your body and let the TSA official wand you but not your pump.

Your Quick-Start "Do" Sheet

Make copies and use this worksheet to begin any "Do" in a way that works best for you. You can download a copy of this worksheet at diabetesbydesign.com/publications.

The "Do" I will do is:

_____

_____

_____

Why it's important to me to do this:

_____

_____

_____

My "How-To" is/are:

_____

_____

_____

When I will begin:

_____

_____

_____

How often I will do this:

_____

_____

_____

Where I will do this:

_____

_____

_____

Who can support me:

_____

_____

_____

What can stop me:

_____

_____

_____

What I will do about that:

_____

_____

_____

What was successful and how I can keep doing it:

_____

_____

_____

For Health Care Professionals: How to Work More Effectively with Patients

You can help empower your patients to adopt healthier behaviors by working with them on the Quick-Start "Do" Worksheets in this book. The worksheets enable patients to more easily take a new action, and they use behavior change strategies that have been proven to be effective. Working with your patients on the worksheet, by using the strategies below, and the questions at the end of this section, will help you to help your patients:

- Focus on what they want (better health) rather than what they don't want (complications)

- Envision a more hopeful future

- Build on what they're already doing well—no matter how small it is

- Discover what they have done successfully in the past and how to apply it here

- Prepare for obstacles and have a plan to overcome them

We know from neuroscience that people are more motivated when they are looking toward what they want, not what they don't want, and that we tend to move in the direction we're looking. For instance, telling someone to lose weight focuses them on the fact that they weigh too much, not on having a slimmer, fitter body. Reminding patients that if they don't do what you say, they may get complications, activates the fear center in the brain, not the part that helps us see possibilities and move enthusiastically toward taking healthier actions. The first "golden rule" is guide patients in the direction you want them to go.

No matter what small things patients are doing well, start there and build on it with small steps forward. For instance, if they're eating two green vegetables a week, congratulate them and see if they can fit in a third. Building on what's working—plus giving patients hope and a picture of an idealized future to work toward, working with positive rather than negative emotions, and helping them recall what's worked in the past to bring to their management now—energizes more sustainable positive actions. Plus, preparing for challenges ensures even greater sustainability.

While part of your work is to teach and inform patients what they need to do to live healthfully with diabetes, we also know that living with a chronic illness, patients need encouragement and support. They do best when they feel you support their efforts without judgment.

We also know that when patients are invited to partner in designing their treatment plan, they are more likely to follow it. In other words, don't only recommend what your patients should do, but also ask open-ended questions that stimulate their thinking around what they want to do, and are willing and feel able to do. Working in collaboration with patients will create a more successful plan—and more successful outcomes for both of you.

Open-ended questions are the opposite of questions to which you answer with one word, like "yes" or "no." They are "thinking questions" that ignite one's mind to search for an answer. Asking open-ended questions of your patients, you may find they come up with answers while working with you, or they may find their answers after they leave. You have switched on their brain, and it will not shut off until it finds an answer.

Here are some suggested open-ended questions to use when you first greet your patients, and when working with them on the worksheet:

• Since we last saw each other, what is going well with your diabetes? What has improved?

• How did you make those improvements?

• What else is working well for you?

• What could we work on that would help you to make tomorrow a little bit better than today?

• On a scale of 1 to 10 in managing your diabetes, where 1 is "I feel I am doing poorly" and 10 is "I am doing the best I can," what grade would you give yourself?

Follow-up questions:

1. Great, what is it that you do that makes it this number?

2. What small step could you take that would make that number half a point higher?

3. How can I help you with that? Who else could help you achieve that?

• Looking at your blood sugar numbers I see many that are in range. Congratulations! How did you do that? How can you do more of that?

• If you were to make just one small improvement, what would that be? Why would this be valuable to you?

• What "Do" from Riva's book would you like to work on? How would it look when you are successful with this "Do"?

• What one or two "How-To's" would you like to use to help you achieve this "Do"?

What Diabetes Is—and Why it's Confusing

The next few pages provide a brief overview of diabetes. You'll understand what diabetes is, how it works in your body, and why the "Do's" and "How-To's" in this book can help you take better care of your diabetes, and yourself, to live your healthiest life.

Very simply, diabetes is a condition where your body has trouble keeping your blood sugar (glucose) within normal range. We all need glucose in our body to function. Glucose gives us energy by fueling our cells and organs, including the brain, heart, and muscles. In a person without diabetes, when glucose rises the body automatically keeps the glucose level within "normal" range by producing insulin. For someone with diabetes, insulin production doesn't work properly and our blood sugar rises and stays above normal unless treated.

There are several types of diabetes. The most common, which you hear about most of the time, is type 2 diabetes. Other types include type 1 diabetes, LADA (latent autoimmune diabetes in adults), gestational diabetes, and MODY (mature onset diabetes in youth). I'm also including pre-diabetes here since it is considered by many to be the first stage of type 2 diabetes.

Type 2 Diabetes

About 90 percent of people who have diabetes have type 2 diabetes. A decade ago, type 2 diabetes was called "Adult Onset" diabetes because mostly adults over the age of fifty got it. But over the last decade, children and younger people have been getting it at an increased rate, tied to the rise in childhood obesity.

If you have type 2 diabetes, your body either doesn't produce enough insulin (the hormone that controls blood sugar) or your body doesn't respond to insulin's effects properly and, therefore, fails to keep your blood sugar in normal range. This is known as insulin-resistance. People who have type 2 diabetes have insulin-resistance. In other words, you are essentially resistant, to some degree, to the insulin your body produces. Without enough insulin, or when you're unable to use insulin properly, your blood sugar rises beyond the normal range and stays there. Too much sugar circulating in your blood, over time, causes damage to your body's organs, large and small blood vessels, and nerves. This damage is known as diabetes complications. Major complications include vision problems, kidney failure, foot ulcers, amputation, nerve damage, digestive issues, stroke, and heart attacks.

How Insulin Works

Insulin is a natural hormone that your body makes in an organ called the pancreas. After you eat or drink, your body breaks down the sugar (glucose) you ingest in your blood stream. Carbohydrate foods turn into the greatest amount of sugar in the blood, much more than protein or fats. Carbohydrate foods are sweets and starches like cake, candy, fruits, milk, sodas, juice, cereal, grains, bread, pasta, potatoes, pretzels, chips, corn, rice, tortillas, cinnamon buns, and chocolate hazelnut frappucinos.

Insulin's job is to keep your blood sugar within normal range. When you don't make enough insulin, or your body is resistant to it, the sugar in your blood rises and stays high and causes you to feel unwell, fatigued, and, over time, causes the damage we call diabetes complications.

Of the nearly 23 million Americans who have type 2 diabetes, about one quarter don't know they have it. How is that possible? Well, you can function for years with high blood sugar and not feel any symptoms. Also, since many people have been living with type 2 diabetes for years when they are diagnosed, about one quarter already have some complications when they are diagnosed.

Symptoms/Risk Factors

Typical symptoms of type 2 diabetes include being very thirsty, peeing a lot, feeling tired, blurry vision, hunger, infections that are slow to heal, and pain, tingling, or numbness in your hands and/or feet.

Although we still don't know what causes type 2 diabetes, researchers have identified several risk factors. These include a family history of diabetes, being overweight, eating a poor diet, getting little to no physical activity, having given birth to a baby weighing over nine pounds, your birth weight being over nine pounds, and/or belonging to a high risk group such as Native American, African American, Hispanic, and Pacific Islander.

Diagnosis

Doctors typically use one of three different blood tests to test for type 2 diabetes. They may use an A1C test, fasting plasma glucose test (FPG), or oral glucose tolerance test (OGTT). People are considered to have type 2 diabetes if:

- their A1C (a measure of average blood sugar over the past two to three months) is higher than 6.5%,

- their FPG (this is a blood test taken in the morning before you eat breakfast) is equal to or over 126 mg/dl (7 mmol/l), or

- their OGTT (your blood sugar is checked before you eat in the morning, then you drink a sugar-rich drink and receive a blood sugar check two hours later) shows your blood sugar two hours after the drink is 200 mg/dl (11.1 mmol/l) or above.

A random blood test for glucose can also indicate type 2 diabetes. A blood glucose greater than or equal to 200 mg/dl (11 mmol/l) is considered diabetes.

Treatment

For people with type 2 diabetes, the usual treatment plan is to lose weight if necessary, eat a healthy diet, get physical activity, manage stress, perhaps take a pill to control blood sugar (most people start on Metformin), and check your blood sugar periodically. Because high blood pressure and high cholesterol often accompany type 2 diabetes, many people are put on prescription medications to keep these in control.

For most people with type 2 diabetes, insulin production weakens over time and/or your body uses the insulin you produce less and less effectively. At this point, your doctor will typically prescribe additional pills or an injectable medicine like Byetta, Victoza, or insulin to control your blood sugar. Almost half of the people with type 2 diabetes will find, over time, that they no longer produce enough insulin, so pills and injectables will no longer control their blood sugar, and they will need to take insulin. There is no shame in using insulin. If your doctor recommends insulin, it is because it is the best medicine to control your blood sugar. What's most important is keeping your blood sugar in your target range as much as possible so you will be less likely to get diabetes complications.

Some people with type 2 diabetes can reduce the amount of medicine they take, or stop taking medicine entirely, by losing a small amount of body weight (five to ten percent), eating healthfully, and being physically active. Not everyone can control type 2 diabetes in this manner (it tends to be more likely if you've been diagnosed within the last few years). That said, eating healthy and being physically active can improve anyone's diabetes and health.

Type 1 Diabetes

Type 1 diabetes is far less common than type 2. Only about 10 percent of people with diabetes have type 1. Type 1 diabetes also used to be called something else, "juvenile diabetes," because it often occurs in children and teenagers. But since adults also get type 1, and children with type 1 grow up to be adults, its name was changed.

Type 1 diabetes has a different cause than type 2 diabetes. It is an autoimmune condition. Ordinarily, our immune system protects our body from viruses and foreign substances. In people with type 1 diabetes, however, their immune system has attacked and destroyed their body's insulin-producing (beta) cells that reside in the pancreas. Scientists don't yet know what causes the body to attack its own beta cells, though they are hard at work trying to figure out why. Right now, scientists believe type 1 diabetes may be caused by a combination of genetic and environmental factors such as toxins or a virus one may have had. Unfortunately, right now, there's nothing a person can do to prevent or avoid getting type 1 diabetes.

People with type 1 diabetes make barely a trace or no insulin so they need to put insulin back into their body. Without it they will die. The only way to put insulin into the body is by injecting it, or by wearing an insulin pump that delivers micro pulses of insulin. This doesn't mean type 1 diabetes is "worse" than type 2, it's just different.

Many symptoms of type 1 diabetes are similar to type 2. They include being very thirsty, peeing a lot, feeling tired, blurry vision, hunger, weight loss, and infections that heal slowly. However, with type 1 diabetes you may have fruity breath if you have ketones (a byproduct of the body burning fat instead of carbohydrates), or lose consciousness.

Diagnosis

Most people with type 1 diabetes are diagnosed with a random blood glucose test and exhibiting the typical symptoms. Doctors may also test for type 1 diabetes in the three common ways they test for type 2 diabetes (see Diagnosis under Type 2 Diabetes). Additional blood tests to indicate type 1 check for proteins in a person's immune system that cause the body to attack itself and for ketones that are often present in the blood and urine of someone with uncontrolled type 1 diabetes.

Treatment

Like type 2 diabetes, being healthy with type 1 diabetes includes maintaining a normal weight, eating healthfully, physical activity, taking insulin and any other medications, checking your blood sugar frequently, and doing your best to reduce stress.

At diagnosis, you will immediately be put on insulin and you will need to take insulin for the rest of your life—or hopefully, until a cure is found. Because you make no insulin—and there's always some element of guessing the exact proper dose based on the carbohydrates you eat, exercise you get, and whether you are stressed or ill—it is important to check your blood sugar frequently. Only by checking frequently can you keep your blood sugar in or near your target range. Your doctor will also tell you what to do when your blood sugar is too high and too low. You will also learn what precautions to take to reduce incidents of low blood sugar, because your blood sugar dropping very low can cause seizures or a loss of consciousness.

As someone living with type 1 diabetes for forty years, I can tell you that by following your treatment plan, you can live a very full and healthy life. I do. In fact, some believe that people who are currently being diagnosed with type 1 diabetes may outlive everyone else because, by following a healthy lifestyle from the start, they will be healthier than the greater population.

LADA

LADA is a form of type 1 diabetes that generally occurs in adults over the age of thirty. People with LADA do not have insulin resistance like people with type 2 diabetes. Like people with type 1, their beta cells are being destroyed, but more slowly. After several years, if you have LADA, you will need to take insulin to control your blood sugar. People with LADA usually do not have a family history of diabetes and are often misdiagnosed with type 2 diabetes. A lab test that shows GAD positive antibodies is used to diagnose LADA, as is a test for C-peptides. Some think LADA is its own form of diabetes, and others say it's just type 1 in adults.

Gestational diabetes

Women who are diagnosed with diabetes during pregnancy have gestational diabetes. Gestational diabetes usually starts mid-way through pregnancy when the hormones a woman's body produces block insulin from doing its job. An oral glucose tolerance test between weeks twenty-four and twenty-eight of pregnancy indicates whether you have gestational diabetes.

Women most at risk for gestational diabetes are older than twenty-five when they get pregnant, have a family history of diabetes, had an unexplained miscarriage or stillbirth before, have already given birth to a baby weighing more than nine pounds, have high blood pressure, and/or are overweight during pregnancy. The symptoms for gestational diabetes are similar to those for type 2 diabetes: being thirsty, peeing a lot, feeling tired, blurry vision, hunger, infections that are slow to heal, and pain, tingling, or numbness in your hands or feet.

Women with gestational diabetes are put on a strict diet, and if necessary, insulin, during pregnancy to manage their blood sugar and minimize risks to the unborn baby. After a woman gives birth, gestational diabetes typically goes away. However, women who get gestational diabetes have a higher risk of developing type 2 diabetes within five to ten years of their pregnancy. Also, babies born to mothers who've had gestational diabetes have a higher risk of developing type 2 diabetes in their lifetime.

MODY

MODY stands for "Maturity Onset Diabetes of the Young." It is a group of rarer forms of diabetes (experts estimate only about 2 percent of people with diabetes have it) caused by the mutation of a gene. MODY tends to occur in people under the age of twenty-five and runs in families. It's thought some thin type 2s may actually have MODY and not type 2 diabetes. Many people with MODY can be treated with pills and/or a healthy, lower-carbohydrate meal plan. Doctors use a blood test for pancreatic antibodies and C-peptide levels to detect MODY, but some say only expensive genetic testing tells whether or not you have MODY for sure.

Pre-diabetes

If your doctor says, "You are borderline," or "You have a touch of sugar," then you have pre-diabetes. Today 80 million people in the United States have pre-diabetes. If you have pre-diabetes, your blood sugars are higher than normal but not as high as the measurement for type 2 diabetes.

The good news about knowing you have pre-diabetes is that by taking healthy actions now (following many of the "Do's" in this book), you can delay or reduce your risk of getting type 2 diabetes. In a landmark study, the Diabetes Prevention Program, people with pre-diabetes reduced or delayed their risk of getting type 2 diabetes by 58 percent. They did this by losing seven to ten percent of their body weight by eating less fat and fewer calories, maintaining 150 minutes of moderate activity a week, and receiving individual counseling. These healthy lifestyle changes worked even better for participants who were sixty years old and older. It reduced their risk of developing type 2 diabetes by 71 percent! Comparatively, people in the control group, who took Metformin (typically the first medication prescribed for patients with type 2 diabetes) and made no other changes, only reduced their risk of developing type 2 diabetes by 31 percent.

Diagnosis

The tests to determine if you have pre-diabetes are the same as the tests for type 2 diabetes. They include an A1C test, fasting plasma glucose test (FPG), or oral glucose tolerance test (OGTT). People are considered to have pre-diabetes if:

- their A1C (a measure of average blood sugar over the past two to three months) is between 5.7% and 6.4%,

- their FPG (this is a blood test taken in the morning before you eat breakfast) is between 100 mg/dl (5.5 mmol/l) and 125 mg/dl (6.9 mmol/l), or

- their OGTT (your blood sugar is checked before you eat in the morning, then you drink a sugar-rich drink and receive a blood sugar check two hours later) shows their blood sugar is between 140 mg/dl (7.7 mmol/l) and 199 mg/dl (11 mmol/l).

Why diabetes is confusing

Diabetes is confusing for a number of reasons, and you are not at fault if you are confused. Now you know there are different types of diabetes that have different names, different causes, and require different treatments.

Also, in the daily care of our diabetes, many different factors affect our blood sugar, blood pressure, and cholesterol, including what we eat, how much we eat, skipping meals, physical activity, our medicines, smoking, stress, and being sick. Yet no one tells us clearly *how* these factors affect our diabetes and what to do about them. In addition, often no one tells us what to do about the numbers that show up on our meters or those we get back from our lab tests.

I don't know of any other disease which we patients are so responsible for managing, yet most of us don't have the information we need to do so. Plus, as if that weren't enough, every day we seem to hear conflicting reports about something related to diabetes. Even scientific findings from trials and studies seem to keep changing.

I hope now with this book you will feel you have what you need to manage your diabetes well. If you want more information about diabetes and pre-diabetes to help you more fully understand the conditions, you'll find it in my book, *50 Diabetes Myths That Can Ruin Your Life and the 50 Diabetes Truths That Can Save It.*

*Your history
doesn't have to be
your future.*

*What counts
is what
you do next.*

*What one small step
can you take today
to live with diabetes
a little better?*

Take it.

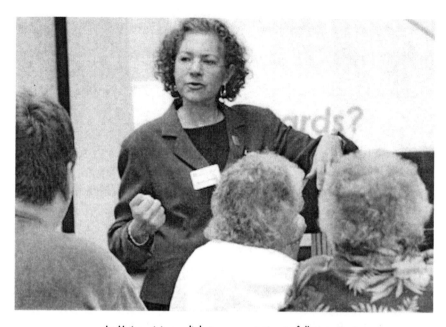

In Maine giving a diabetes presentation to fellow patients.

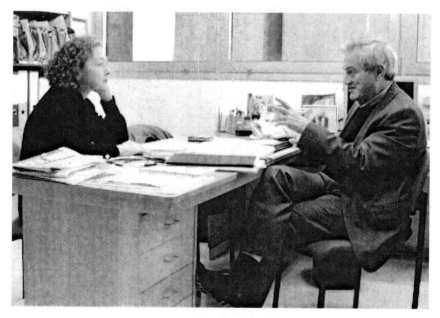

Learning from renowned diabetologist Professor Itamar Raz in Israel.

Postscript

This is my third book. At times it was a bear to write, but I am so grateful it now exists. It is so essential that we know how to take care of our diabetes, and ourselves. This book is also part of what I've been working toward for a few years, four books that together will give you everything you need to live your healthiest, happiest life with diabetes.

I wrote my first book, *The ABCs Of Loving Yourself With Diabetes*, from pure passion. An introspective kid, I've always been interested in how we see ourselves and the world, and how we keep on keepin' on—which is something you have to do with diabetes. This book guides you to develop the emotional strength to weather the ups and downs of diabetes, the storms that come and go, and to also treat yourself more kindly and gently, with more forgiveness and patience. I still go back and read a few pages from time to time and they continue to inspire me.

Then I wrote my second book, *50 Diabetes Myths That Can Ruin Your Life and the 50 Diabetes Truths That Can Save It*, because what you need to live well with diabetes—in addition to emotional resilience—is to know what diabetes is, to understand why it works the way it does, and to know how to work it.

The fourth book is the one I've been working on for some time and will finish next year. It's about flourishing with diabetes. As I've been saying for a while now, you can have a great life not *despite* having diabetes, but *because* of it.

From where I sit now that completes the set. You will have a guide for staying emotionally strong, the understanding of diabetes and how to manage it, the clear and simple actions steps to manage it, and the path toward creating a life with diabetes that is vibrant and rich with possibilities.

Stay tuned.

Recommended Websites (in alphabetical order)

American Diabetes Association (diabetes.org)
ASweetLife.org
BehavioralDiabetesInstitute.org
ChildrenwithDiabetes.com
CloseConcerns.com
dLife.com
DiabetesDaily.com
DiabetesFamilies.com
Fit4D.com
Insulindependence.org
JDRF.org
Joslin.org
MayoClinic.com
Mendosa.com
QuantiaMD.com
WebMD.com

Social Communities

DiabetesSisters.org (female-specific)
DiabeticConnect.com
MyGlu.org (Type 1 diabetes-specific)
Juvenation.org (Type 1 diabetes-specific)
PatientsLikeMe.com
TuDiabetes.org

Acknowledgments

You may have heard the expression, "It takes a village." In other words, it takes a community to create something. This book took a village. And while my name is on the cover, making these pages my sole responsibility (including errors or critical omissions), this book was only possible due to the contribution of others.

In truth when I began, I had little idea how the research and writing process would unfold, and less idea who would help me unfold it. Yet with no promises of gold or diamonds, not even a nice dinner, an amazing group of colleagues came to my side just with my asking, "Would you help?" They said yes even though their plate was full or, for some, overflowing. They made time even when it meant giving away gorgeous spring weekends. They all have my deepest gratitude.

My thank you's go to Kathy Spain. I first met Kathy when she came to New York City some years ago for a JDRF scientific conference. She invited me to meet her for a drink in lower Manhattan. It was dark, it was pouring rain, and I was tired. I argued with my lazy self about whether to go. Luckily, my responsible self won and I went. Kathy was my right hand on this book, as she was on my previous book, *50 Diabetes Myths That Can Ruin Your Life and the 50 Diabetes Truths That Can Save It.*

To Lynda Schultz Sardeson, who in addition to everything else she does, each year goes to Africa to give of herself and her expertise at local clinics. From that, you know Lynda would never say no to me, and she never has. To Susan Weiner, who in the middle of her crazy schedule made time for me, no questions asked, and I went back to the well again and again. To Sandy Merrill, whom I met through a mutual friend, and over lunch we joyously broke down the nutritional value of every morsel we ate, much to the dismay of our dining companion. To Delaine Wright, whose endless zest, passion, and desire for her patients to succeed gave me endless smiles. To Michael Dansinger, who was only too happy to help me get this book into your hands. I am indebted to him for his unwavering support.

To my many gentle, and nudging, readers: Gretchen Becker, Regina Berezovskaya, Claire Blum, Constance Brown-Riggs, Wil Dubois, Scott Johnson, Margaret Moore, Heather Nielsen, Alyssa Rosenzweig, Janis Roszler, Wendy Satin Rapaport, Betsy Snell, Hope Warshaw, Carol Weber, and anyone I may have unintentionally left out, my sincerest apologies, you all made this book better. To my friends and acquaintances who readily supplied me with their tips, photos, and shots of encouragement (yes, pun) to keep moving forward.

To Claire Gerus, my literary agent, who when I started poured me countless cups of white tea. From the time she introduced herself to me on the phone on a cold winter's night, Claire has been, and continues to be, my trusted ear and well of encouragement. To Bill Greaves, my book designer, who went above and beyond again and again to please me and who is an incredible artist in his own right. To Gary Feit, my editor, who made this whole book better, not just as an editor, but also with the wealth of knowledge he brought, and whose hands I felt completely safe in.

To Haidee Merritt, single panel illustrator, whose talent I admire and whose cartoons make me laugh. Whether she had just come in from gardening or was straining her eyes over a drawing, Haidee was always ready to help, to make it work, to share this ride. Some of my most fun email exchanges during the days and nights when this felt like tough going were with Haidee.

And to Boudewijn Bertsch, my husband, partner, and friend, who owes me a major blow-out dinner with the folding of this book. There would be no book, as well as so many other things that make my life so joyful, without you.

About the Author

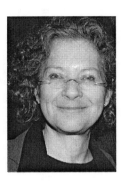

Riva Greenberg is a diabetes patient-expert and health coach who has lived successfully with type 1 diabetes for forty years, since the age of eighteen. Author of two previous diabetes books, *50 Diabetes Myths That Can Ruin Your Life and the 50 Diabetes Truths That Can Save It* and *The ABCs Of Loving Yourself With Diabetes*, Riva writes about diabetes and health on *The Huffington Post* and on a blog on her website, DiabetesStories.com.

She is an inspirational speaker at conferences, health fairs, hospitals, and corporations, and conducts workshops on flourishing with diabetes. She knows first-hand that we can live an exceptional life, not *despite* having diabetes but *because* of it. She also helps medical professionals work more effectively with patients, particularly regarding behavior change.

Riva is among the top ten diabetes online influencers, and advises medical device and pharmaceutical companies. She has also been inspiring patients since 2007 as a peer-mentor. She is a an advisory member of the Diabetes Hands Foundation and a member of the American Association of Diabetes Educators and Diabetes Advocates.

Finally, she doesn't know why authors always write where they live, but in keeping with literary tradition, she lives in Brooklyn.

To contact Riva to speak to, or give a workshop for, patients or providers, please write to her at DiabetesbyDesign.com/contact.

About the Artist

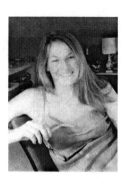

Haidee Soule Merritt is an author and illustrator who has most recently focused her talents on capturing life with diabetes in black and white images. Her cartoons express day-to-day impressions that can be both subtle and unsettling, but almost always amusing.

A veteran of the disease for almost forty years, Haidee is using her experiences and unique voice to spread an understanding of the disease to a broader audience.

Haidee studied English and Classics at Franklin & Marshall College and the University of Washington, and resides now in the seacoast town of Portsmouth, New Hampshire. More samples of her work and musings can be found on her website, HaideeMerritt.com.

Glossary

A1C: *See* Hemoglobin A1c.

Basal: The fasting state. Basal insulins are long-acting insulins that prevent blood sugar from rising in between meals.

Beta cells: Cells in the pancreas that produce insulin and secrete it into the blood stream.

Blood pressure: The pressure exerted by circulating blood against the walls of blood vessels. Blood pressure is recorded as two numbers—the systolic pressure (as the heart beats) over the diastolic pressure (as the heart relaxes between beats). The measurement is written one above or before the other, with the systolic number on top and the diastolic number on the bottom.

Body mass index (BMI): A number calculated from a person's weight and height that provides an indicator of body fatness and is used to determine potential health risks.

Bolus: The insulin used at mealtimes to cover carbohydrates and keep blood sugar levels normal.

Cannula: A flexible plastic tube attached to an insulin pump with a small needle at the end that is inserted through the skin into the top layer of fatty tissue to deliver a constant drip of insulin.

Carbohydrate: One of the major food groups, including simple sugars and more complex starches. Carbohydrates are the body's main energy source and are the nutrients that most raise blood sugar. Also referred to as "carb."

Celiac disease: A digestive disease that damages the small intestine and interferes with absorption of nutrients from food. People who have celiac disease cannot tolerate gluten, a protein in wheat, rye, and barley. Linked to type 1 diabetes because both are auto-immune conditions.

Complex carbohydrate: Made from longer, more complex chains of sugar than simple carbohydrates. These are digested more slowly, and raise blood sugar less rapidly, than simple carbohydrates.

Diabetes: *See* type 1 diabetes; type 2 diabetes; gestational diabetes.

Fasting blood glucose (sugar): The blood sugar value before the first meal of the day.

Fat: A source of calories and energy in food that is highest in calories. Fat does not directly raise blood sugar and can slow the rise of blood sugar when consumed with carbohydrates.

Foot ulcer: An open sore on the foot that can either be a shallow crater involving only the surface skin or extend through the full thickness of the skin, involving tendons, bones, and other deep structures. Foot ulcers are the most common cause of lower extremity amputation.

Gastroparesis: A neuropathy, nerve damage, that is caused by prolonged high blood sugar and in which the stomach is slow to empty its contents. This causes blood sugar after meals to be unpredictable. Also called delayed stomach emptying.

Gestational diabetes: A condition in which women without previously diagnosed diabetes exhibit high blood glucose levels during pregnancy. A diagnosis of gestational diabetes is a risk marker for developing type 2 diabetes.

Glucagon: A hormone that is produced by the pancreas and causes blood sugar to rise.

Glucagon emergency kit: A small kit available at pharmacies and consisting of an injectable that releases the body's stored glucose in order to raise blood sugar quickly when a patient is experiencing severe hypoglycemia and is unable to eat carbohydrates.

Glucose: Sugar in the blood stream.

Glycogen: A starchy substance that is formed from glucose and is made by, and stored in, the liver and muscles. It can rapidly be converted into glucose.

Hashimoto's disease: An auto-immune disorder resulting from the immune system attacking the thyroid gland. The inflammation caused by Hashimoto's disease most often leads to an under-active thyroid gland (hypothyroidism).

HDL: The "good" cholesterol. High-density lipoprotein, a particle that is found in the blood and is believed to offer protection from coronary artery disease.

Hemoglobin A1c: A blood value that reflects average blood glucose for the past two to three months. The Hemoglobin A1c (A1C) test measures what percentage of a person's hemoglobin—a protein in red blood cells that carries oxygen—is coated with sugar.

Hyperglycemia: Abnormally high blood sugar.

Hypertension: High blood pressure.

Hypoglycemia: Abnormally low blood sugar, defined as blood sugar below 70 mg/dl (3.9 mmol/l).

Hypoglycemic unawareness: Inability to experience or perceive the physical symptoms of abnormally low blood sugar.

Insulin: A hormone that is produced by the beta cells in the pancreas and facilitates the entry of glucose into most cells in the body.

Insulin-resistance: Reduced sensitivity to insulin's effect on blood sugar, either because the pancreas does not produce enough insulin or because the body does not use insulin effectively. Associated with obesity.

Ketoacidosis: An acute, life-threatening condition that is caused by hyperglycemia and dehydration and that affects people with type 1 diabetes. Ketoacidosis causes ketone production and acidification of the blood.

Ketone: Fat deposits produced when fatty acids are broken down for energy.

Latent autoimmune diabetes in adults (LADA): A genetically linked, hereditary auto-immune disorder that causes the body to mistake the pancreas as foreign and to respond by attacking and destroying the insulin-producing beta islet cells of the pancreas.

LDL: The "bad" cholesterol. Low-density lipoprotein, a particle in the blood that deposits cholesterol and triglycerides in arterial walls. Elevated LDL is a risk factor for coronary artery disease and peripheral vascular disease.

Lipid: A fat or fat-like substance found in the blood, such as cholesterol.

Macrovascular: Related to large blood vessels in the body.

mg/dl: Milligrams per deciliter, the unit in which blood sugar is measured in the United States.

Microvascular: Related to small blood vessels in the body.

mmol/l: Millimoles per liter, the unit in which blood sugar is measured outside of the United States (1 mmol/l = 18 mg/dl).

Nephropathy: A complication of diabetes due to elevated blood glucose that causes kidney damage and disease.

Neuropathy: Nerve damage, a complication of diabetes due to elevated blood glucose.

Oral glucose tolerance test: Measures the body's ability to use glucose, the body's main source of energy. Usually performed in the morning after several hours' fast, this test consists of drinking a glucose-rich solution and drawing blood two hours afterward to measure glucose levels.

Oral medication: Pills used to lower blood glucose in type 2 diabetes.

Pancreas: An abdominal organ that manufactures and secretes insulin, glucagon, and other hormones and enzymes into the blood stream.

Peripheral neuropathy: A complication of diabetes that causes nerve damage resulting in pain, typically described as tingling, burning, or numbness in the hands and feet.

Postprandial: After a meal; typically refers to a blood test taken two hours after beginning a meal.

Pre-diabetes: An abnormal state of high glucose that raises a person's risk of developing type 2 diabetes, heart disease, and stroke. Once referred to as "borderline" diabetes.

Retinopathy: Injury to the retina, the light-sensing surface in the back of the eye. Usually caused by chronically high blood sugars.

Simple carbohydrate: A carbohydrate that can be rapidly converted to glucose by the digestive process. Also called simple sugar.

Sulfonylureas: A class of oral glucose-lowering medications that stimulate beta cells to produce more insulin.

Triglycerides: Fats found in blood and fatty tissues. Elevated triglycerides, which are often the result of elevated blood sugar, are a risk factor for vascular disease.

Type 1 diabetes: One of the two major types of diabetes, characterized by a total or near total loss of the capacity to produce insulin. Affects youth in larger numbers than adults. Previously called juvenile diabetes.

Type 2 diabetes: The most common type of diabetes, characterized by partial loss of insulin-producing capability and/or resistance to the effect of insulin. Usually appearing after age forty-five, although increasing in children. Commonly associated with overweight, obesity, and being sedentary. Previously called adult-onset diabetes.

Vascular disease: Any condition that affects your circulatory system. This ranges from diseases of your arteries, veins, and lymph vessels to blood disorders that affect circulation.

References

Come to the Edge
Rees, Nigel. *Cassell Companion to Quotations,* London, UK: Cassell, 1997.

Food Note
Apple, Jessica. "Carbs Or Fat: What Really Makes Us Gain Weight?" 2012. DiabetesMine.com. <http://www.diabetesmine.com/2012/04/carbs-or-fat-what-really-makes-us-gain-weight.html>.

Dietary Intake of Saturated Fat By Food Source and Incident Cardiovascular Disease: The Multi-Ethnic Study of Atherosclerosis, 2012. <http://www.ncbi.nlm.nih.gov/pubmed/22760560>.

Micozzi, Dr., Another Outdated Verse in the Gospel of Government Guidelines, 2012. <http://drmicozzi.com/another-outdated-verse-in-the-gospel-of-government-guidelines>.

Do #1. Say "Bye-Bye" to Diets
"Overeating: Why Willpower is Not Enough." 7/11. RD411.com. <http://www.rd411.com/index.php?option=com_content&view=article&id=5093:overeating-why-willpower-is-not-enough&catid=136:weight-control&Itemid=424>.

Wells, Alyssa. "Organize Your Mind for Weight Loss Success." 2012. fitbie. *Rodale Inc.* <http://fitbie.msn.com/lose-weight/tips/organize-your-mind-weight-loss-success/tip/0>.

Ianzito, Christina. "Fat Chance!" *AARP, The Magazine.* 2012.

Kathleen M Zelman, MPH, RD, LD. "Lose Weight, Gain Tons of Benefits." Web MD. <http://www.webmd.com/diet/features/lose-weight-gain-tons-of-benefits>.

Goldman, Leslie. "The New Health Rules; You'll Like Them Better Than the Old Ones, We Promise." *O Magazine.* page 102. 2012.

Melnick, Meredith. "Studies: Why Diet Sodas Are No Benefit to Dieters." 2011. *Time Healthland.* <http://healthland.time.com/2011/06/29/studies-why-diet-sodas-are-no-boon-to-dieters/>.

Wolpert, Stuart. "UCLA Researchers Find That People Who Lose Weight Usually Gain it All Back—Plus Some." 2007. *UCLA Magazine.* UCLA. <http://www.magazine.ucla.edu/exclusives/dieting_no-go/>.

Traci Mann, A. Janet Tomiyama, Erika Westling, Ann-Marie Lew, Barbra Samuels, and Jason Chatman. "Medicare's Search for Effective Obesity Treatments: Diets Are Not the Answer." University of California, Los Angeles. <http://motivatedandfit.com/wp-content/uploads/2010/03/Diets_dont_work.pdf>.

Do #2. Seek Health First from Your Foods

David B Agus, *The End of Illness,* (1 edn, Free Press, 2012): pp. 158–173.

Buff, Sheila. "Nix the Nonfat Milk, Chuck the Lowfat Cheese? (Continued)." 2012. dLife.com. <http://www.dlife.com/diabetes-food-and-fitness/what_do_i_eat/fats/non-fat.page01>.

"10 Worst and Best Foods." *Nutrition Action.* Center for Science in the Public Interest. <http://www.cspinet.org/nah/10foods_bad.html>.

Mark Hyman, MD. "Eat Your Medicine: Food as Pharmacology." *The Huffington Post.* <http://www.huffingtonpost.com/dr-mark-hyman/food-as-medicine_b_1011805.html>.

Dr. Susan Mitchell, PhD, RD, FADA. "Just a Spoonful of Sugar…How Much is Too Much?" 2009. <http://www.susanmitchell.org/blog/2009/08/just-a-spoonful-of-sugar…how-much-is-too-much/>.

Shaw, Gina. "Soda and Osteoporosis: Is There a Connection?" WebMD. <http://www.webmd.com/osteoporosis/features/soda-osteoporosis>.

Andriani, Lynn. "6 New Superfoods You Definitely Haven't Tried Before." 2012. <http://www.oprah.com/food/Superfoods-List-2012-Sunchokes-Adzuki-Beans-Chia-Seed>.

Kulas, Michelle. "How Often Should You Eat Sweets?" 2011. *LiveStrong.* <http://www.livestrong.com/article/491653-how-often-should-you-eat-sweets/>.

Robin Wulffson, MD. "Artificial Sweeteners May be a Healthy Choice." 2012. Emax Health. <http://www.emaxhealth.com/11306/artificial-sweeteners-may-be-healthy-choice>.

Hurlock, Stephen Perrine with Heather. "15 New Superfoods." *Men's Health.* <http://www.menshealth.com/mhlists/New_American_Diet_Superfoods/>.

"Turmeric Component Reduces Type 2 Diabetes Incidence." 2012. Diabetes In Control.com. <http://www.diabetesincontrol.com/index.php?option=com_content&view=article&id=13166&catid=1&Itemid=17>.

Do #3. Make Your Kitchen a Shrine to Heart Health
"Fish and Omega-3 Fatty Acids." 2010. American Heart Association. <http://www.heart.org/HEARTORG/GettingHealthy/NutritionCenter/HealthyDietGoals/Fish-and-Omega-3-Fatty-Acids_UCM_303248_Article.jsp>.

"Healthy Dietary Fats; The Truth About Fat, Nutrition, and Cholesterol." HELPGUIDE.org. <http://helpguide.org/life/healthy_diet_fats.htm>.

"Diet and Lifestyle Recommendations." American Heart Association. <http://www.americanheart.org/presenter.jhtml?identifier=851>.

"Diabetes Awareness Month." The Heart of Diabetes. American Heart Association. <http://www.iknowdiabetes.org/diabetes-awareness-month.html>.

Dietary Intake of Saturated Fat By Food Source and Incident Cardiovascular Disease: The Multi-Ethnic Study of Atherosclerosis. 2012. <http://www.ncbi.nlm.nih.gov/pubmed/22760560>.

"5 Medication-Free Strategies to Help Prevent Heart Disease." 2010. mayoclinic.com. <http://www.mayoclinic.com/health/heart-disease-prevention/WO00041>.

Davis, Jeanie Lerche. "25 Top Heart-Healthy Foods: These 25 Foods Are Loaded With Heart-Healthy Nutrients That Help Protect Your Cardiovascular System." Web MD. <http://www.webmd.com/food-recipes/features/25-top-heart-healthy-foods>.

Huget, Jennifer Larue, "Chicken Skin: Good for You After All." 2010. <http://www.healthzone.ca/health/dietfitness/diet/article/788197-chicken-skin-good-for-you-after-all>.

Jegtvig, Shereen. "Ten Foods for a Healthy Heart." 2008. About.com. <http://nutrition.about.com/od/foodfun/a/healthy_heart.htm>.

Do #4. Toss a Rainbow on Your Plate
"How Many Fruits & Vegetables Do You Need?" CDC. <http://www.fruitsandveggiesmatter.gov/>.

"Glycemic Index Food Chart." *South Beach Diet.* <http://www.southbeach-diet-plan.com/glycemicfoodchart.htm>.

Laino, Charlene. "Fruit May Protect Against Diabetes Eye Problems." 2012. WebMD. <http://www.webmd.com/eye-health/news/20120614/fruit-and-diabetic-retinopathy>.

Spero, David. "Vegetables to the Rescue." 2012. <http://www.diabetesselfmanagement.com/Blog/David-Spero/vegetables-to-the-rescue/?ref=ls>.

Webber, Roxanne. "How Many Fruits and Vegetables Should I Eat: A Visual Guide." 2011. CHOW. <http://www.chow.com/food-news/80652/how-many-fruits-and-vegetables-should-i-eat-a-visual-guide/>.

Jegtvig, Shereen. "What is a Serving of Fruit or a Vegetable?" 2012. About.com. <http://nutrition.about.com/od/fruitsandvegetables/f/servingfruit.htm>.

Do #5. Get "the Skinny" on Fat

"Questioning Carbohydrate Restriction in Diabetes Management." 2012. Issue 626. Diabetes In Control.com. <http://www.diabetesincontrol.com/index.php?option=com_content&view=article&id=12814&catid=1&Itemid=17>.

"Friendly Fats—and Fiendish Ones." 2010. cbs news. <http://www.cbsnews.com/stories/2010/06/10/earlyshow/health/main6567619.shtml?tag=cbsnewsTwoColUpperPromoArea>.

Peterson, Jan. "Salad Dressing Choices: Which Are Best When Dieting?" 2010. Yahoo Voices! <http://voices.yahoo.com/salad-dressing-choices-which-best-dieting-5374421.html?cat=5>.

Apple, Jessica. "Carbs Or Fat: What Really Makes Us Gain Weight?" 2012. <http://www.diabetesmine.com/2012/04/carbs-or-fat-what-really-makes-us-gain-weight.html>.

Do #6. Keep Your Body Glowing with "Good" Fats

"Study: Light Canned Tuna Has Less Mercury Than White Tuna." 2010. thedailygreen. GoodHousekeeping.com. <http://www.thedailygreen.com/healthy-eating/eat-safe/mercury-in-tuna>.

"Healthy Dietary Fats; The Truth About Fat, Nutrition, and Cholesterol." HELPGUIDE.org. <http://helpguide.org/life/healthy_diet_fats.htm>.

"High Blood Pressure (Hypertension)." American Diabetes Association. <http://www.diabetes.org/living-with-diabetes/complications/high-blood-pressure-hypertension.html>.

Murray, Jennifer. "Sources and Benefits of Healthy Fats." 2009. suite 101.com. <http://proteins-carb-fats.suite101.com/article.cfm/sources_and_benefits_of_healthy_fats>.

Goldman, Leslie. "The New Health Rules; You'll Like Them Better Than the Old Ones, We Promise." *O Magazine.* page 102. 2012.

Teicholz, Nina. "What if Bad Fat is Actually Good for You?" 2007. *Men's Health.* <http://www.menshealth.com/health/saturated-fat/page/3>.

Feinman, Richard. "What if Saturated Fat is Not the Problem?" 2011. dLife. <http://www.dlife.com/diabetes-food-and-fitness/what_do_i_eat/fats/what_if_saturated_fat_not_problem>.

Heller, Samantha. *Get Smart, Samantha Heller's Nutrition Prescription for Boosting Brain Power and Optimizing Total Body Health.* 2010.

Do #7. Shun "Made for Diabetics" Foods

"Reese's Peanut Butter Cups." Hershey's. <http://www.hersheys.com/reeses/products/reeses-peanut-butter-cups/milk-chocolate.aspx>.

"A Sugar-Free Chocolate Reference Guide From Diabetes Health." 2006. *Diabetes Health* magazine/Kings Publishing. <http://www.diabeteshealth.com/media/pdfs/Chocolate-Chart-02-06.pdf>.

Wolfenden, Elizabeth M. "The Nutrition of Sugar Free Reese's." 2010. Livestrong.com. <http://www.livestrong.com/article/330618-the-nutrition-of-sugar-free-reeses/>.

Do #8. Have Less Maybe "Scary Dairy"

"Know Your Fats." 2012. American Heart Association. <http://www.heart.org/HEARTORG/Conditions/Cholesterol/PreventionTreatmentofHighCholesterol/Know-Your-Fats_UCM_305628_Article.jsp>.

Buff, Sheila. "Nix the Nonfat Milk, Chuck the Lowfat Cheese?" 2011. dLife.com. <http://www.dlife.com/diabetes-food-and-fitness/what_do_i_eat/fats/non-fat>.

Buff, Sheila. "Nix the Nonfat Milk, Chuck the Lowfat Cheese? (Continued)." 2012. dLife.com. <http://www.dlife.com/diabetes-food-and-fitness/what_do_i_eat/fats/non-fat.page01>.

"Dietary Intake of Saturated Fat By Food Source and Incident Cardiovascular Disease: The Multi-Ethnic Study of Atherosclerosis." 2012. <http://www.ncbi.nlm.nih.gov/pubmed/22760560>.

"Fat Sources: List of Food High in Total Fat and Saturated Fatty Acids (Beef, Pork, Chicken)." www.dietaryfiberfood.com. <http://www.dietaryfiberfood.com/fat-saturated.php>.

Oz, Dr. Mehmet. "How Much Dairy Should I Eat Per Day?" Share Care. <http://www.sharecare.com/question/how-much-dairy-eat-day>.

Hyman, Dr. Mark. *The Blood Sugar Solution*, Little, Brown and Company, 2012.

Kathryn Flynn, MPH. "Nutritional Differences in Rice, Soy & Almond Milk." 2011. Livestrong.com. <http://www.livestrong.com/article/348025-nutritional-differences-in-rice-soy-almond-milk/>.

Dolson, Laura. "Carbohydrate Counts of Dairy Products." 2007. About.com. <http://lowcarbdiets.about.com/od/whattoeat/a/dairycarbs.htm>.

Beers, Tanya. "Best-Tasting Low-Fat Cheeses." 2006. *Prevention*. Rodale. <http://www.prevention.com/health/weight-loss/eat-to-lose-weight/low-fat-cheese-6-tasty-and-healthy-cheeses/article/7806d08f88803110VgnVCM200 00012281eac__/>.

Do #9. Rethink Your Love Affair with Salt

"Let's Break it Down." *Diabetic Living*. Vol 9, No. 2, page 76 (2012)

"Tips for Lowering Sodium." Cleveland Clinic. <http://my.clevelandclinic.org/disorders/diabetes_mellitus/hic_tips_for_lowering_sodium_for_people_with_diabetes.aspx>.

"Sodium (Salt Or Sodium Chloride)." American Heart Association. <http://www.americanheart.org/presenter.jhtml?identifier=4708>.

Do #10. Fall Madly in Love with Complex Carbs

"Carbohydrates." Centers for Disease Control and Prevention. <http://www.cdc.gov/nutrition/everyone/basics/carbs.html#Simple%20Carbohydrates>.

"Glycemic Index Foods At Breakfast Can Control Blood Sugar Throughout the Day." 2012. The Institute of Food Technologists. <http://www.ift.org/newsroom/news-releases/2012/march/30/glycemic-index.aspx>.

"How to Choose Good Carbs When Food Shopping." *Reader's Digest*. <http://www.rd.com/health/good-carbs-shopping-for-better-nutrition/>.

Spero, David. "Stop Spiking Those Sugars!" 2012. *Diabetes Self-Management*. <http://www.diabetesselfmanagement.com/Blog/Blood-Glucose-Monitoring/stop-spiking-those-sugars/?ref=ls>.

Spero, David. "Beans Will Rock Your World." 2012. *Diabetes Self-Management.* <http://www.diabetesselfmanagement.com/Blog/David-Spero/beans-will-rock-your-world/?ref=ls>.

Spero, David. "Glycemic Index Confusion." 2012. *Diabetes Self-Management.* <http://www.diabetesselfmanagement.com/Blog/David-Spero/glycemic-index-confusion/?ref=ls>.

Do #11. Turn Ho-Hum Oatmeal into Your "Can't-Wait-For" Breakfast
"Recipe: Overnight Crock Pot Oatmeal." 2010. Frugal Upstate.com. <http://www.frugalupstate.com/recipes/recipe-overnight-crock-pot-oatmeal/>.

Do #12. Fill Your Shopping Cart with Farm-Fresh Foods
Pollan, Michael. *Food Rules: An Eater's Manual.* 2010. Penguin Books.

Do #13. Become a Label Maven: Check Carbohydrates, Fat, Sodium, and Fiber
"Basic Carbohydrate Counting: What is Carbohydrate Counting?" 2012. Drugs.com. <http://www.drugs.com/cg/basic-carbohydrate-counting.html>.

Strauch, Ingrid. "How Do You Do Fiber?" 2009. *Diabetes Self-Management.* <http://www.diabetesselfmanagement.com/Blog/Ingrid-Strauch/how_do_you_do_fiber/>.

Dolson, Laura. "Sugar's Many Disguises: Recognizing Sugar on Food Labels." About.com. <http://lowcarbdiets.about.com/od/whattoeat/a/sugars.htm>.

Terry, Sarah. "Low Carb Diet and Chocolate." 2011. Livestrong.com. <http://www.livestrong.com/article/375839-low-carb-diet-and-chocolate/>.

Do #14. Graze—It's Good for You!
"Heart and Vascular Health & Prevention, Small Meals and Cholesterol." ClevelandClinic.com. <http://my.clevelandclinic.org/heart/prevention/askdietician/ask4_02.aspx>.

"Advantages of Eating Small Meals Throughout the Day." Helium.com. <http://www.helium.com/items/1808524-advantages-of-eating-small-meals-through-the-day>.

Diane Welland, MS, RD. "Living the Clean Life." 2009. *Today's Dietitian.* <http://www.todaysdietitian.com/newarchives/111609p42.shtml>.

Do #15. When Drinking, Keep Your Blood Sugar from Sinking

Megrette Fletcher M.Ed, RD, CDE. "What Will Alcohol Do to My Blood Sugar?" 2012. Diabetes and Mindful Eating.com. <http://www.diabetes andmindfuleating.com/>.

Do #16. Eat From 9-Inch Dinner Plates

"Change Plates, Lose Weight" Health.com. <http://diet.health.com/2009/01/16/ change-plates-lose-weight/>.

"Use Smaller Plates to Get Big Weight-Loss Benefits." Health.com. <http:// www.health.com/health/article/0,20409972,00.html>.

Brian, PhD., Wansink, *Mindless Eating.* Psych Central. <http://psychcentral .com/lib/2011/mindless-eating/>.

Do #18. Keep a Food Diary and Double Your Weight Loss

"CHR Study Finds Keeping Food Diaries Doubles Weight Loss." 2008. The Center for Health Research. <http://www.kpchr.org/research/public/News .aspx?NewsID=3>.

"Food Diary Doubles Weight Loss." 2008. *emPower Magazine.* <http://www .empowernewsmag.com/listings.php?article=58>.

"Nutrition: Keeping a Food Diary." FamilyDoctor.org. <http://familydoctor .org/online/famdocen/home/healthy/food/general-nutrition/299.html>.

Christ, Scott. "Food Journal Analysis." eHow. <http://www.ehow.com/ how_4447482_keep-food-diary.html>.

Neithercott, Tracey. "Recording What You Eat Can Help With Blood Glucose Control and Weight." *Diabetes Forecast.* American Diabetes Association. <http://forecast.diabetes.org/magazine/food-thought/keeping-a-food-journal>.

Do #19. Stay on Track Despite Holiday Temptations

"10 Surprising Ways to Avoid Weight Gain During the Holidays." 2008. *US News.* <http://health.usnews.com/health-news/blogs/on-women/2008/12/02/10- surprising-ways-to-avoid-weight-gain-during-the-holidays>.

"8 Steps to Surviving Holiday Weight Gain." 11/09. Cleveland Clinic. <http:// my.clevelandclinic.org/heart/prevention/nutrition/holidayeating12_01.aspx>.

Do #20. Limit Fast Food—Or You'll Be "Fat Fast!"

"24 Surprisingly Healthy Fast Foods." 2012. FitnessMagazine.com. Meredith Corporation. <http://www.fitnessmagazine.com/recipes/healthy-eating/ on-the-go/healthy-fast-foods/?page=3>.

Greenberg, Riva. "Dr. Michael Roizen: 'You Can't Make a Deal With Food'." 08/11/10. *The Huffington Post.* <http://www.huffingtonpost.com/riva-greenberg/dr-michael-roizen-you-can_b_677538.html>.

El-Buri, Hend. "Nutritional Values of Starbucks Drinks." 2010. Livestrong.com. <http://www.livestrong.com/article/260294-nutritional-values-of-starbucks-drinks/>.

"That Grande Mocha Frappuccino Can Add Up the Calories." KOMO Staff & News Services. <http://www.komonews.com/news/archive/4128051.html>.

Steven, PhD., Aldana, "The Stop & Go Fast Food Nutrition Guide." 2008. *The Stop & Go Fast Food Nutrition Guide.* Maple Mountain Press. <http://www.bc.com/corporate/BCWellnessProgram/Nutrition/mainContent/0/text_files/file1/Fast%20Food%20Guide.pdf>.

Wilder, Andrew. "Healthy Options At Subway." 2010. eatingrules.com. <http://www.eatingrules.com/2010/05/healthy-options-at-subway/>.

Do #21. Learn Your "Diabetes A-B-C's"

"Heart and Vascular Health & Prevention." Cleveland Clinic. <http://my.clevelandclinic.org/heart/prevention/cholesterol/cholesterolguidelines9_01.aspx>.

"Liposcience Finds Success in Numbers." NC State University. <http://ncsu.edu/research/results/vol6/6.html>.

Davis, Jeanie Lerche. "Supplementing Your Heart Health: Omega-3, Plant Sterols, and More." WebMD. <http://www.webmd.com/vitamins-and-supplements/lifestyle-guide-11/supplementing-your-heart-health-omega-3-plant-sterols>.

Do #22. Know How to Delay or Prevent Diabetes Complications

"Checking Your Blood Glucose." American Diabetes Association. <http://www.diabetes.org/living-with-diabetes/treatment-and-care/blood-glucose-control/checking-your-blood-glucose.html>.

Wong, Cathy. "What is Alpha Lipoic Acid?" 2011. About.com. <http://altmedicine.about.com/od/alphalipoicacid/a/alphalipoicacid.htm>.

Dropeski, Kathy. "Target Blood Glucose Levels for Diabetics." 2011. Livestrong.com. <http://www.livestrong.com/article/364899-target-blood-glucose-levels-for-diabetics/>.

Do #24. Take a Peek at Your Feet

"Peripheral Arterial Disease." American Diabetes Association. <http://www.diabetes.org/living-with-diabetes/complications/peripheral-arterial-disease.html>.

Dubois, Wil. "Ask D'mine: All About Seizures, and Cold Funky Feet." 2012. DiabetesMine.com. <http://www.diabetesmine.com/2012/08/ask-dmine-all-about-seizures-and-cold-funky-feet.html#more-55733>.

Malaskovitz, PhD, RN, CDE, Joyce and Susan Rush Michael, DNSc, RN, CDE. "When Your Legs Ache." 2009. *Diabetes Self Management.* <http://www.diabetesselfmanagement.com/articles/diabetic-complications/when-your-legs-ache/>.

Wong, Cathy. "What is Alpha Lipoic Acid?" 2011. About.com. <http://altmedicine.about.com/od/alphalipoicacid/a/alphalipoicacid.htm>.

Do #25. Get Thee to an Ophthalmologist or Optometrist

"Facts About Diabetic Retinopathy." 2009. National Eye Institute. <http://www.nei.nih.gov/health/diabetic/retinopathy.asp>.

Do #27. Have a Sick Plan Before You Get Sick

"Sick Days and Diabetes." BD Diabetes. <http://www.bd.com/us/diabetes/page.aspx?cat=7001&id=7347>.

"Living With Diabetes Ketoacidosis (DKA)." American Diabetes Association. <http://www.diabetes.org/living-with-diabetes/complications/ketoacidosis-dka.html>.

Do #28. Know What to Expect Before You're Expecting

"Prenatal Care." American Diabetes Association. <http://www.diabetes.org/living-with-diabetes/complications/pregnant-women/prenatal-care.html>.

"Sick-Day Guidelines for People With Diabetes Causes, Symptoms and Treatment." 2010. Everyday Heatlh Inc. <http://www.everyday-health.com/health-center/sick-day-guidelines-for-people-with-diabetes.aspx?xid=tw_diabetesfacts_20111214_sickday>.

Do #29. Seek Treatment if Your Sex Drive Has Taken the Off Ramp

"Erectile Dysfunction and Diabetes." 2011. WebMD. <http://www.webmd.com/erectile-dysfunction/guide/ed-diabetes>.

Feldman, H.A., Goldstein, I., Hatzichristou, D.G., Krane, R.J., McKinley, J.B. "Sexual Dysfunction and Diabetes." Joslin Diabetes Center. <http://www.joslin.org/info/sexual_dysfunction_and_diabetes.html>.

Dubois, Wil. "Men's Health: Between the Ears or Below the Beltline?" 2012. DiabetesMine.com. <http://www.diabetesmine.com/2012/06/mens-health-between-the-ears-or-below-the-beltline.html>.

Do #30. Give Up Smoking if You Smoke

"About Chantix." Chantix. <http://www.chantix.com/about-chantix.aspx>.

"Nicotine Can Raise A1C By 34 Percent." Diabetes In Control.com. <http://www.diabetesincontrol.com/articles/diabetes-news/10741-nicotine-can-raise-a1c-by-34-percent>.

Do #32. Winterize Yourself Against the Flu

"If You Have Diabetes, a Flu Shot Could Save Your Life." CDC. <http://www.cdc.gov/diabetes/projects/pdfs/eng_brochure.pdf>.

Manning, Anita. "Flu Vaccine Myths, Misconceptions." 2006. *USA Today.* <http://www.usatoday.com/news/health/2006-09-25-flu-myths_x.htm>.

Do #33. Know How to Inject if You Inject

"How to Inject Insulin." BD Diabetes. <http://www.bd.com/us/diabetes/page.aspx?cat=7001&id=7257>.

"How to Inject Insulin With a Syringe or Insulin Pen." Islets of Hope. <http://www.isletsofhope.com/diabetes/treatment/insulin_inject_1.html>.

Do #35. Be Prepared for Hypoglycemia

"Hypoglycemia (Low Blood Glucose)." American Diabetes Association. <http://www.diabetes.org/living-with-diabetes/treatment-and-care/blood-glucose-control/hypoglycemia-low-blood.html>.

"Hypoglycemia (Low Blood Sugar) in People Without Diabetes—Topic Overview." 2011. WebMD. <http://diabetes.webmd.com/tc/hypoglycemia-low-blood-sugar-topic-overview>.

Scheiner MS, CDE, Gary. "Exorcising the Specter of Nighttime Hypoglycemia." 2012. *Diabetes Self-Management.* <http://www.diabetesselfmanagement.com/articles/low-blood-glucose/exorcising-the-specter-of-nighttime-hypoglycemia/?ref=ls/>.

Do #36. Know if Weight-Loss Surgery Is an Option for You
Campbell, Amy. "Weighty Matters: What's New in the Weight-Control Arena." 2012. *Diabetes Self-Management.* <http://www.diabetesselfmanagement.com/Blog/Amy-Campbell/weighty-matters-whats-new-in-the-weight-control-arena/?ref=ls>.

Erika, PhD., Gebel. "Weight-Loss Surgery and Type 2 Diabetes: Is Bariatric Surgery a Shortcut to a 'Cure'?" *Diabetes Forecast.* American Diabetes Association. <http://forecast.diabetes.org/magazine/features/weight-loss-surgery-and-type-2-diabetes>.

"Study Finds Diabetes Can Recur in Some After Weight Loss Surgery." 2012. Mayo Clinic. <http://www.mayoclinic.org/news2012-sct/6959.html>.

Do #39. Bring Your Doctor These Questions
"Make Your Doctor Visits Count." BD Update. (2010).

Do #41. Understand that Exercise Is Medicine
"Ketoacidosis (DKA)." American Diabetes Association. <http://www.diabetes.org/living-with-diabetes/complications/ketoacidosis-dka.html>.

"A Guide for Adults 55 and Up." 2011. Living Health with Diabetes. American Diabetes Association. <http://www.diabetes.org/assets/pdfs/living-healthy-with-diabetes-guide.pdf>.

"After Your Workout Continue to Check Your BG." 2012. A Sweet Life.org. <http://asweetlife.org/a-sweet-life-staff/tips/exercise-tips/when-your-workout-is-over-dont-stop-check-your-bg/26475/>.

"Do's and Don'ts of Exercise for Diabetics." 2008. Yahoo. <http://voices.yahoo.com/dos-donts-exercise-diabetics-850027.html?cat=5>.

Do #42. Realize Exercise Doesn't Need a Special Outfit
Lukach, Mark. "Best Standing Desks." 2012. The Wirecutter. <http://thewirecutter.com/reviews/best-standing-desks/>.

Do #45. Start with a Single Step and Aim for 10,000 a Day
"Getting Started on the 10,000 Steps Program." Shape up America!. <http://www.shapeup.org/shape/steps.php>.

"The Verdict is in: Moderate Exercise Improves Insulin Sensitivity." BD Update. (2010).

Cheng, Jacqui. "How the Fitbit Got Me to Walk More and be Part of Society Again." 2012. *Conde Nast.* <http://arstechnica.com/staff/forcequit/2012/04/how-the-fitbit-got-me-to-walk-more-and-be-part-of-society.ars>.

Do #46. Plan To Be the Next "Biggest Winner"
"AACE: Reality Weight-Loss TV Meets Medical Skeptics Over Exercise." Diabetes in Control. <http://www.diabetesincontrol.com/articles/diabetes-news/12877-aace-reality-weight-loss-tv-meets-medical-skeptics-over-exercise>.

Waehner, Paige, "What is Vigorous Exercise?" 2012. <http://exercise.about.com/od/cardioworkouts/a/Vigorous-Exercise.htm>.

Do #47. Do Some Heavy Breathing and Heavy Lifting
"Will Pumping Iron Fight Dementia?" 2010. NHS choices. <http://www.nhs.uk/news/2010/01January/Pages/Will-pumping-iron-fight-dementia.aspx>.

Fiore, Kristina. "Exercise Benefit in Diabetes Upheld." 2012. Medpage Today Everyday Health. <http://www.medpagetoday.com/Endocrinology/Diabetes/34077>.

Hanson, Chad L. "The Case for Combined Training." *The Sport Digest*—ISSN: 1558-6448. United States Sports Academy <http://thesportdigest.com/archive/article/case-combined-training>.

Oz, Dr. Mehmet. "Dr. Oz's 7 Reasons to Start Building Muscle Today A Beginner's Guide to Building Healthy Muscles—And Lengthening Your Life." *O Magazine.* Oprah Winfrey. <http://www.oprah.com/health/Building-Healthy-Muscles-How-to-Build-Muscle-Dr-Oz>.

Do #48. Respect Your Mother, but Go Ahead and Fidget
Agus, David. "Running to Sit Still," *The End of Illness.* 2011.Free Press, a division of Simon & Schuster: pp. 229–232.

Do #50. De-stress and De-compress
Biermann, Sarah. "Interview With Dr. Jill Bolte Taylor." 2008. Sarah Biermann's Blog. <http://imagicreation.wordpress.com/2008/05/05/interview-with-dr-jill-bolte-taylor/>.

Do #51. Shut Down with Plenty of Shut-Eye
"Sleep Apnea Treatment May Improve Diabetes." 2005. WebMD. <http://diabetes.webmd.com/news/20050301/sleep-apnea-treatment-may-improve-diabetes>.

Mann, Denise. "Can Better Sleep Mean Catching Fewer Colds? Lack of Sleep Affects Your Immune System." WebMD. <http://www.webmd.com/sleep-disorders/excessive-sleepiness-10/immune-system-lack-of-sleep?page=2>.

McGonigal Ph.D, Kelly, "The Science of Willpower. Secrets for Self-Control Without Suffering." 2011. *Psychology Today.* <http://www.psychologytoday.com/blog/the-science-willpower/201107/the-neurobiology-dont-shop-when-youre-hungry>.

Do #52. Exercise Your Brain: Be in Learning Mode

"Top 25 Diabetes Blogs." Blog Rank.com. <http://www.invesp.com/blog-rank/Diabetes>.

Do #55. Aim for Better, Not Perfect

Polonsky, Bill. "Taking a Diabetes Vacation." The Emotional Side Of Diabetes: 10 Things You Need To Know. Behavioral Diabetes Institute. <http://behavioraldiabetesinstitute.org/downloads/brochure-Diabetes-10-Things-To-Know.pdf>.

Nathaniel G. MD, MS, RD, Clark. "Defending ADA's A1C Target." Doc News. ADA. <http://docnews.diabetesjournals.org/content/2/10/3.full>.

Do #59. Develop a Personal Support Network

"Good Friends Can Keep You Healthy." 2011. ThirdAge.com. <http://www.thirdage.com/friendship/good-friends-can-keep-you-healthy>.

Greenberg, Riva. "Build Your Personal Support Network." QuantiaCare. <https://eatsmart.quantiacare.com/>.

Parker-Pope, Tara. "Go Easy on Yourself, a New Wave of Research Urges." 2011. *New York Times.* <http://well.blogs.nytimes.com/2011/02/28/go-easy-on-yourself-a-new-wave-of-research-urges/>.

Do #60. Make "I'm Grateful" a Daily Mantra

Fabrega, Marelisa. "How Gratitude Can Change Your Life." <http://www.thechangeblog.com/gratitude/>.

Robert, Ph.D., Brooks. "Gratitude and Kindness: Small Gestures, Large Impact." <http://www.drrobertbrooks.com/writings/articles/1204.html>.

Bonus Do's
1. Make a Citizen's Arrest if You Have "Diabetes Police" in Your Life

Polonsky, Bill. "Arresting the Diabetes Police." The Emotional Side of Diabetes: 10 Things You Need to Know. Behavioral Diabetes Institute. <http://behavioraldiabetesinstitute.org/downloads/brochure-Diabetes-10-Things-To-Know.pdf>.

4. Know How To Get Medicines and Supplies Covered if Money is Tight

"Health & Drug Plans." <http://www.medicare.gov/default.aspx>.

"Financial Help for Diabetes Care." National Diabetes Information Clearinghouse. National Institute of Diabetes and Digestive and Kidney Diseases (NIDDK), National Institutes of Health (NIH). <http://diabetes. niddk.nih.gov/dm/pubs/financialhelp/>.

"Participating Patient Assistance Programs." Partnership for Prescription Assistance. <http://www.pparx.org/en/prescription_assistance_programs/ list_of_participating_programs>.

Walmart Rolls Out Lower Prices on Diabetes Supplies. *Diabetes Self-Management.* July 28, 2012. <http://www.diabetesselfmanagement.com/Blog/ Web-Team/walmart-rolls-out-lower-prices-on-diabetes-supplies/?ref=ls>.

5. Travel Smart and Travel Safe

"Hidden Disabilities Travelers With Disabilities and Medical Conditions." Transportation Security Administration. <http://www.tsa.gov/travelers/airtravel/ specialneeds/editorial_1374.shtm#3>.

What Diabetes Is—and Why it's Confusing

"What is Diabetes." JDRF. <http://www.jdrf.org/index.cfm?page_id=101982>.

"What is Diabetes?" IDF Diabetes Atlas. International Diabetes Federation. <http://www.idf.org/diabetesatlas/5e/what-is-diabetes>.

"Prediabetes FAQS." American Diabetes Assocation. <http://www.diabetes. org/diabetes-basics/prevention/pre-diabetes/pre-diabetes-faqs.html>.

"Diabetes Prevention Program." 2011. NIH Publication No. 09-5099 October 2008. National Diabetes Information Clearinghouse (NDIC). <http:// diabetes.niddk.nih.gov/dm/pubs/preventionprogram/#results>.

Porter, Dr. John. "What is MODY?" 2008. Children with Diabetes.com. <http://www.childrenwithdiabetes.com/clinic/mody.htm>.

Ruhl, Jenny, "A Rare Form of 'Type 1.5' That is Often Misdiagnosed." <http:// www.phlaunt.com/diabetes/14047009.php>.

The following books have also informed my research and thinking:

Agus, David B. *The End of Illness,* (1 edn, Free Press, 2012): pp. 158–173

Bernstein, Richard K. Dr. *Bernstein's Diabetes Solution: The Complete Guide to Achieving Normal Blood Sugars* (4 Rev Upd edn, Little, Brown and Company, 2011).

Covey, Stephen R. *The 7 Habits of Highly Effective People* (Revised edn, Free Press, 2004).

Deutschman, Alan. *Change Or Die: The Three Keys to Change At Work and in Life* (HarperBusiness, 2007).

Duhigg, Charles. *The Power of Habit: Why We Do What We Do in Life and Business* (1 edn, Random House, 2012).

Greenberg, Riva. *The ABCs of Loving Yourself With Diabetes* (SPI Management LLC, 2007).

Greenberg, Riva. *50 Diabetes Myths That Can Ruin Your Life And the 50 Diabetes Truths That Can Save It* (1 Original edn, Da Capo Lifelong Books, 2009).

Halvorson, Heidi Grant. *Nine Things Successful People Do Differently* (Harvard Business Review Press, 2011).

Halvorson, Heidi Grant. *Succeed: How We Can Reach Our Goals* (Reprint edn, Plume, 2011).

Hyman, Mark. *The Blood Sugar Solution: The Ultrahealthy Program for Losing Weight, Preventing Disease, and Feeling Great Now!* (1 edn, Little, Brown and Company, 2012).

Kabat-Zinn, Jon. *Full Catastrophe Living: Using the Wisdom of Your Body and Mind to Face Stress, Pain, and Illness* (First Edition edn, Delta, 1990).

Kegan, Robert, and Laskow Lahey, Lisa. *Immunity to Change: How to Overcome it and Unlock the Potential in Yourself and Your Organization* (Leadership for the Common Good) (1 edn, Harvard Business School Press, 2009).

Kessler, David A. *The End of Overeating: Taking Control of the Insatiable American Appetite* (Reprint edn, Rodale Books, 2010).

Lieberman, David J. *How to Change Anybody: Proven Techniques to Reshape Anyone's Attitude, Behavior, Feelings, or Beliefs* (St. Martin's Griffin, 2005).

Ornish, Dean M.D. *The Spectrum: A Scientifically Proven Program to Feel Better, Live Longer, Lose Weight, and Gain Health* (Pap/DVD Re edn, Ballantine Books, 2008).

Maurer, Robert. *One Small Step Can Change Your Life: The Kaizen Way* (Workman Publishing Company, 2004).

May, Michelle, M.D. *Eat What You Love, Love What You Eat With Diabetes: A Mindful Eating Program for Thriving With Prediabetes or Diabetes* (1 edn, New Harbinger Publications, 2012).

Moore, Margaret, and Hammerness, Paul. *Organize Your Mind, Organize Your Life: Train Your Brain to Get More Done in Less Time* (Original edn, Harlequin, 2011).

Ofri, Danielle. *Incidental Findings: Lessons From My Patients in the Art of Medicine* (1 edn, Beacon Press, 2006).

Patterson, Kerry, Joseph Grenny, David Maxfield, Ron McMillan, and Al Switzler. *Change Anything: The New Science of Personal Success* (Reprint edn, Business Plus, 2012).

Pollan, Michael. *Food Rules: An Eater's Manual* (Penguin Books, 2010).

Polonsky, William H. *Diabetes Burnout: What to Do When You Can't Take it Anymore* (1 edn, American Diabetes Association, 1999).

Prochaska, James O., John Norcross, and Carlo DiClemente. *Changing for Good: A Revolutionary Six-Stage Program for Overcoming Bad Habits and Moving Your Life Positively Forward.* (William Morrow Paperbacks, 1995).

Remen, Rachel Naomi. *Kitchen Table Wisdom: Stories That Heal* (Edition Unstated edn, Riverhead Trade, 1997).

Seligman, Martin E. P. *Authentic Happiness: Using the New Positive Psychology to Realize Your Potential for Lasting Fulfillment* (Free Press, 2004).

Sisson, Mark. *The Primal Blueprint: Reprogram Your Genes for Effortless Weight Loss, Vibrant Health, and Boundless Energy* (Primal Blueprint Series) (2 edn, Primal Nutrition, Inc., 2012).

Sweet, Victoria. *God's Hotel: A Doctor, a Hospital, and a Pilgrimage to the Heart of Medicine* (1 edn, Riverhead Hardcover, 2012).

Weber, Doron. *Immortal Bird: A Family Memoir* (1 edn, Simon & Schuster, 2012).

CPSIA information can be obtained at www.ICGtesting.com
Printed in the USA
LVOW121804150513

333966LV00022B/979/P